P9-CRR-089

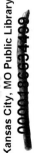
Kansas City, MO Public Library
0001863440

Living Well with
Hemochromatosis

A Healthy Diet for Reducing Iron Intake, Managing Symptoms, and Feeling Great

Anna Khesin, RD, CDN

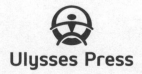

Ulysses Press

Text copyright © 2019 Anna Khesin. Design and concept copyright © 2019 Ulysses Press and its licensors. All rights reserved. Any unauthorized duplication in whole or in part or dissemination of this edition by any means (including but not limited to photocopying, electronic devices, digital versions, and the internet) will be prosecuted to the fullest extent of the law.

Published in the United States by:
Ulysses Press
P.O. Box 3440
Berkeley, CA 94703
www.ulyssespress.com

ISBN: 978-1-61243-901-3
Library of Congress Catalog Number: 2018967980

Printed in Canada by Marquis Book Printing
10 9 8 7 6 5 4 3 2 1

Acquisitions editor: Casie Vogel
Managing editor: Claire Chun
Project editor: Renee Rutledge
Proofreader: Susan Lang
Front cover and interior design: what!design @ whatweb.com
Cover photo: © Elena Eryomenko/shutterstock.com
Production: Jake Flaherty

IMPORTANT NOTE TO READERS: This book has been written and published for informational and educational purposes only. It is not intended to serve as medical advice or to be any form of medical treatment. You should always consult with your physician before altering or changing any aspect of your medical treatment. Do not stop or change any prescription medications without the guidance and advice of your physician. Any use of the information in this book is made on the reader's good judgment and is the reader's sole responsibility. This book is not intended to diagnose or treat any medical condition and is not a substitute for a physician. This book is independently authored and published and no sponsorship or endorsement of this book by, and no affiliation with, any trademarked brands or other products mentioned within is claimed or suggested. All trademarks that appear in ingredient lists and elsewhere in this book belong to their respective owners and are used here for informational purposes only. The author and publisher encourage readers to patronize the quality brands mentioned in this book.

Contents

Chapter 8

Recipes 45

Introduction

Chances are, you have many questions about hemochromatosis. For the following real people, the quest for answers began with unexplained symptoms.

"Lucy," at 46 years old, was experiencing weakness, lethargy, joint pain, and difficulty walking. She had stopped menstruating approximately two years prior and developed hot flashes around that time.[1]

Danny, a gay man, feared that he may have been exposed to HIV after he developed a persistent, itchy rash.[2]

Rick persistently consulted with a variety of doctors to attempt to determine the cause for his fatigue, gray skin hue, hair loss, and severe pain in the abdomen as well as in a couple of fingers and knuckles.[3]

Darryl, despite leading a healthy lifestyle, encountered advancing symptoms over the span of two decades, beginning at age 34. His initial reason for concern was his elevated triglycerides along with an intensifying pain in the knees, hips, and big toe. Eventually, the joint pain only worsened, and feelings of exhaustion were perpetual. In his forties, Darryl began to experience irregular heartbeat, weight gain, bloating,

---

1. L. Rojas-Roldan and T. Wilkins, "Case Report," *The Journal of Family Practice* 66, no. 6 (2014): 305–308.
2. P. Whitaker, "Health Matters," *New Statesman* (2015): 63.
3. Canadian Hemochromatosis Society. "Iron Chronicles: Rick." Accessed June 30, 2018, https://www.toomuchiron.ca/iron-chronicles/rick/.

abdominal pain, and depression. By his fifties, he was diagnosed with sleep apnea and was found to have uncontrollable blood sugar.[4]

What could all of these symptoms mean? No one story is identical to the other. Those who experience them could be male, female, homosexual, heterosexual. Danny's itchy skin could be the outcome of an iron deficiency. Rick could just be a hypochondriac, always anxious over the slightest discomfort, running back to the doctor with a new discovery alongside the same old complaints. And Darryl could simply be experiencing the typical signs of aging. It's not uncommon to have less energy or to put on a little weight over the years. For his high triglycerides, he began to be treated with medication once diet intervention and exercise proved to be unsuccessful. The joint pain was considered to be gout, wear and tear from years of running, and the beginnings of arthritis. These are all seemingly unrelated symptoms. Could there possibly be a common thread?

The simple answer is yes. A condition by the name of hemochromatosis, if undetected, can compromise vital organs in the body, which can result in widespread symptoms and diseases. The silver lining in all of this is, if you have decided to read this book, then you likely either already know that you have the disorder or know someone who does and can now go on a path toward health and longevity.

This book is intended to offer insight into what hemochromatosis is and how the foods that you eat can contribute to the burden or can help manage it better with the help of a collection of simple and delicious recipes. Most importantly, this book was written to impart useful tips so that you are empowered to confidently venture out and enjoy meals other than the ones provided in this guide.

---

4. Canadian Hemochromatosis Society. "Iron Chronicles: Darryl." Accessed June 30, 2018, https://www.toomuchiron.ca/iron-chronicles/darryl/.

Chapter 1

What Is Hemochromatosis?

Hemochromatosis is a hereditary condition that causes the body to absorb and store too much iron. (For the purposes of this book, I will use the terms "hemochromatosis" and "hereditary hemochromatosis" interchangeably.) Being that it is inherited and therefore rooted in one's genes, it is not a disorder that is contagious or can one day randomly appear. All people have an HFE gene (think "H" stands for hereditary, and "Fe" is the symbol for iron on the periodic table), which plays a key role in tightly regulating iron metabolism in the body. If this gene is mutated, hereditary hemochromatosis may develop. A variety of mutations are possible, some more closely associated with the development of hemochromatosis than others. Researchers are continuously discovering variant mutations of the HFE gene, allowing us to have greater insight into the disease.

The three most common mutations that precipitate hemochromatosis are C282Y, H63D, and S65C. The C282Y type is the one most commonly found in people whose bodies are unable to regulate iron absorption.

In order to have hemochromatosis, a person needs to receive two copies of the defective gene—one from their father and one from their mother. However, having both copies does not automatically mean that iron overload will develop. It simply indicates that there is increased risk. The chances are greater in individuals who have two copies of the C282Y mutation than those with one C282Y mutation and one copy of the H63D or S65C mutation.

Those who have only one copy of the mutated gene are considered to be carriers. They can pass along this mutation to their children and likely will not experience hemochromatosis themselves unless they also have another mutation that enhances iron absorption. Whether or not their child will inherit hemochromatosis depends on the makeup of the other parent's HFE gene. Since the presence of hemochromatosis is dependent on a person's family tree, anyone diagnosed should proactively share their story with blood relatives and encourage them to get tested.

Under normal circumstances, the body carefully regulates the absorption of iron. If body stores are low, absorption is enhanced. If stores are high, then absorption is diminished. Typically, only 8% to 10% of the iron from foods is absorbed. The remaining 90% passes through and gets taken up by cells in the intestinal tract, where it eventually dies and is excreted through fecal matter. Only small amounts of absorbed iron are eliminated through blood loss, sweat, urine, and the shedding of cells from the skin and gastrointestinal tract. In hemochromatosis, the absorption rate increases up to fourfold and continues at this rate even when the body is overloaded.

This is a trend that starts at birth and over the years iron amasses to a degree that begins to take a major toll on the body. With all of this iron being absorbed without a way to be excreted, the iron begins to deposit into the organs, joints, and skin. Over time, these organ systems become compromised with the development of organ dysfunction and disease, such as diabetes. If misdiagnosed and improperly treated, the organs may fail, which may result in premature death.

The good news is that with timely diagnosis and proper treatment, the outcome need not be dire. The key is to work closely with your physician to determine which treatment route is best suited for you. The primary form of treatment should then be accompanied by a close look at current dietary and lifestyle habits to determine where modifications need to be made. While you cannot rely on diet alone to manage hemochromatosis, it is an essential part of the equation. The body's exposure to iron is primarily from food. Knowing which foods aid and inhibit the absorption of iron is imperative. Fortunately, a hemochromatosis-friendly diet is all about mindfulness and is nothing extreme.

Chapter 2

Symptoms and Impact on Organ Systems

It is estimated that 1 million Americans have hemochromatosis and roughly 10% of the population in the United States carry the mutated gene. This data translates to hemochromatosis being the primary reason behind iron overload disorder and the leading hereditary disease in individuals of Northern European descent. The Genetic and Rare Diseases Information Center (GARD) makes it a point to highlight that hemochromatosis is not a rare disease. Then why is it that many have never heard of this condition? Why is it so often misdiagnosed and untreated? These are important questions considering that it can be easily diagnosed and managed. When interventions are put in place, individuals can maintain a good quality of life with normal life expectancy.

The answers often lie in symptoms only gradually coming to surface and most often in midlife. Usually, symptoms become more obvious between the ages of 40 and 60. Individual experience with the disorder also varies, with symptoms ranging from mild to severe. To complicate matters further, hemochromatosis can impact various parts of the body, and most of the signs and symptoms can point in the direction of other ailments. Often, they are so unspecific that they are attributed to aging and poor lifestyle habits. For example, fatigue and joint pain are some of the earliest complaints mentioned to doctors, but these can be due to a host of other reasons.

The following lists some of the many signs and symptoms that individuals living with hemochromatosis have reported or were noted to have:

- Chronic fatigue
- Joint pain/swelling/stiffness/disease
- Stomach pain
- Abdominal fluid buildup and swelling
- Impotence
- Amenorrhea (untimely absence of menstruation)
- Lack of sperm in the semen
- Testicular atrophy
- Decline in libido
- Hair loss
- Arrhythmia (irregular heartbeat)
- Enlarged heart
- Changes in skin color
- Elevated blood sugar
- Enlarged liver
- Weight loss or gain
- Increased triglyceride levels
- Thyroid dysfunction
- Changes in mood/personality

Let's now take a closer look at what some of our major organ systems are responsible for and how an overload of iron can lead to complications.

Iron and the Liver

Unlike certain organs such as the appendix, which we can live without, the liver is indispensable. It is a workhorse of an organ that is responsible for hundreds of tasks that are crucial in our day-to-day functioning. One such task is to filter blood coming from both the heart and the intestines. Harmful substances such as ammonia from protein metabolism, drugs, and alcohol are converted into nontoxic by-products that can be safely excreted or reabsorbed by the body.

Not only is the liver a center for detoxification, but it also stores some of the body's fuel for when energy is needed. Following a meal, the intestines supply the liver with blood that is rich in fats, sugars, and vitamins. The liver then releases sugar in the form of glucose back into the bloodstream to be used as energy. Any unused excess glucose is then converted into glycogen and stored in the liver for future use.

The liver produces hepatocytes, cells that help produce and regulate the body's cholesterol levels. This affects production of cholesterol-dependent sex hormones like testosterone and estrogen. Bile produced by the liver is essential in the digestion of fat as well as the absorption of fat-soluble vitamins (vitamins A, D, E, and K). By aiding in the absorption of vitamin K (a key component in the formation of vitamin K–dependent coagulation factors), the liver plays an important role in blood clotting. The liver even houses defense cells that combat bacteria and infections that may have entered the gastrointestinal tract.

Hepcidin, a key iron-regulatory hormone produced predominantly by the liver, helps decrease iron levels in the blood. In a state of iron deficiency, hepcidin is muted so that the body can increase its absorption of iron. When there is an abundance of iron, hepcidin production ramps up. This mechanism is vital because without adequate iron, red blood cells are unable to carry oxygen throughout the body as iron is the backbone of hemoglobin (a protein in red blood cells that is responsible for transporting oxygen in the blood).

The liver also has the capacity to store iron in the form of the protein ferritin. As ferritin, iron is readily available when the body needs to create new red blood cells. Once the capacity of the ferritin molecules is exceeded, iron gets transformed into hemosiderin, another way in which the liver is able to store iron. The problem with large amounts of hemosiderin collecting in an organ like the liver is that it begins to impact the ability of the organ to work properly.

The HFE gene regulates the production of hepcidin. When the HFE gene is mutated due to hereditary hemochromatosis, it is unable to effectively communicate with hepcidin, causing a disruption in the regulation of iron. Excessive iron in the liver can cause the organ to become enlarged and scar tissue to develop (when the scarring is severe it is referred to as cirrhosis). However, iron overload is not the only cause of liver scarring. Alcoholism, viral hepatitis, nonalcoholic steatohepatitis (NASH), and copper overload are a few other conditions that can lead to cirrhosis. Symptoms of cirrhosis include fatigue, stomach pain, fluid accumulation in the legs and abdomen, itching, confusion, and jaundice (yellowing of the skin and whites of the eyes). An overloaded and scarred liver increases the risk of developing liver cancer by as much as two hundredfold.

Iron and the Pancreas

The pancreas has two distinct roles in the body: aiding in digestion of food and regulating blood sugar levels. Partially digested food from the stomach passes into a part of the small intestine known as the duodenum. During this step of the digestive process, the pancreas secretes a clear liquid, which is a mixture of water, sodium bicarbonate, and digestive enzymes. Sodium bicarbonate neutralizes the acidic juice from the stomach that has mixed into the partly digested food. The various enzymes then break down proteins, carbohydrates, and fats into usable nutrients.

The pancreas is intricately involved in the regulation of blood sugar through the production and secretion of hormones. Two of the main hormones, insulin and glucagon, are secreted by the pancreas directly into the bloodstream. They work together to ensure that blood glucose levels don't surge too high (hyperglycemia) or drop too low (hypoglycemia). Following a meal, blood sugar levels rise and insulin is released. Insulin acts like a key to unlock cells, which allows them to take in the sugar for use as energy or to be put into storage. This is critical to well-being since, without being shuffled into appropriate cells, the sugar in the blood will enter vulnerable vessels of the eyes, kidneys, and nerves. With time, irreversible damage to these parts of the body can occur. These effects can be seen in individuals with poorly controlled diabetes who suffer from kidney failure, blindness, and neuropathy.

Glucagon manages the other end of the spectrum, low blood sugar. Repercussions of hypoglycemia range from generalized confusion to seizures, unconsciousness, and death. When levels are low, glucagon signals the body's cells and liver to release stored sugar into the bloodstream. This leads to rapid increases in blood glucose levels in times of need.

Both insulin and glucagon are produced in the area of the pancreas known as the islets of Langerhans. This structure is composed of different types of cells, one type being beta cells (ß-cells). These cells' primary job is to create and eject insulin when necessary. ß-cells require iron for proper functioning; however, in excess it can destroy these cells. For this reason, just like the liver, the pancreatic ß-cells can also create hepcidin to regulate iron levels. Unfortunately, the nature of hereditary hemochromatosis does not allow for such a mechanism to work. Upon the destruction of the ß-cells, glucose homeostasis is disrupted, and diabetes can ensue.

Iron and the Heart

One organ whose purpose most people are familiar with is the heart. Made up of two sides, it is a muscle that directs blood throughout the body. The right side pumps blood to the lungs for oxygen and the left side receives the oxygen-rich blood from the lungs, which then gets pushed out for the body's use. Considering the heart's job, it is clear that iron is needed here. Remember, iron ensures that red blood cells are carrying oxygen. Therefore, either a deficiency or an overload of iron will jeopardize cardiac health. Despite this understanding, all facets of the relationship between iron and car-diovascular disease are still not entirely clear.

What we do know is that under normal circumstances, transferrin, a protein that transports iron, is roughly 30% saturated with iron. In hemochromatosis it is completely saturated, and thus iron circu-lates unbound to this protein. In an unbound state the iron builds up in the cells of the heart muscle, becoming a catalyst for oxidative stress. This sparks a reaction that leads to cell injury and, poten-tially, heart failure.

In heart failure, symptoms like difficulty breathing due to fluid accumulation in the lungs, fatigue, and swelling in the stomach and ankles are common. These symptoms arise from a decline in the heart's pumping ability. Some individuals experience abnormal and irregular heartbeats because the iron has gotten in the way of the conduction of electrical impulses. If the arrhythmia impacts the top chambers of the heart, it can increase chances of having a stroke. Arrhythmias within the lower chambers of the heart are more ominous since the heart can unexpectedly stop beating.

Iron and the Skin

Making up one-sixth of our body weight, the skin is one of our biggest and heaviest organs. To the naked eye it may appear to simply be the body's cover, keeping our internal organs in while keeping external elements like water and bacteria out. Although there is truth to this observation, there is also a lot more to this organ. Made up of three layers—epidermis (outer layer), dermis (middle layer), and hypodermis (lower layer)—the skin is able to carry out functions to protect inner organs and tissues, regulate body temperature, and process physical sensations.

The outer layer consists of dead skin cells (keratinocytes) that shed and get replaced every four weeks. This is one small way in which the body excretes a little bit of iron, with roughly 20% to 25% of absorbed iron excreted in the shedding of keratinocytes. One of these cells' main functions is to prevent the intrusion of dangerous microbes. Any germs that successfully penetrate are then confronted with lymphocytes and Langerhans cells, which help carry these invaders to the lymphatic system for destruction. Other cells present in the epidermis are melanocytes and Merkel cells. The melanocytes generate a dark pigment, melanin, which offers protection from the sun. The greater the exposure to sunlight the more melanin is produced, leading to tanning of the skin. A person's potential for melanin production is directed by their genetics, which is why some people are able to develop a deeper tan while others are more susceptible to redness. Meanwhile, Merkel cells are near nerve endings and respond to pressure, allowing us to feel touch.

The dermis consists of sensory cells and a web of collagen that contributes to the skin's elasticity and strength. This middle layer also houses sweat glands and blood vessels, which are responsible for thermoregulation. When hot, the vessels expand, heat from the blood is let out through the skin, and sweat is released onto the surface of the skin. Under cold conditions, the vessels constrict in an attempt to conserve warmth. Sweat is another vehicle for iron loss but the amount is insignificant.

Best known for its composition of fat and connective tissue, the hypodermis protects bones and joints and insulates the body. This is also the layer of the skin that produces vitamin D in the presence of sunlight.

In hemochromatosis, changes to the skin may be observed. One classic symptom is a change in the skin's pigment. It may look bronzed, metallic, or gray. This hyperpigmentation can take place throughout the body but may be more prevalent in the skin of the face, neck, genital area, and lower portion of the forearms and legs. Iron deposits as well as the excessive iron damaging certain structures within the skin lead to this unusually high production of melanin. Often, areas exposed to the sun have a more pronounced change in color since sunlight stimulates the production of melanin further.

Hereditary hemochromatosis is traditionally taught to medical students as "bronze diabetes," a name first used by Armand Trousseau in 1865 after he detected a connection between diabetes and bronzed skin. In fact, if you dissect the word "hemochromatosis," you get blood (hemo), color/pigment (chromat-), and abnormal condition (-osis).

Hemochromatosis may cause porphyria cutanea tarda (PCT) to develop. PCT is an iron-dependent skin disorder in which blisters surface on areas of the skin exposed to the sun, most often the hands and face. This disease arises from poorly functioning or an inadequate amount of the liver enzyme uroporphyrinogen decarboxylase (UROD). This is problematic because the UROD enzyme is needed to metabolize porphyrins for heme synthesis. Hemes are a part of various proteins, like hemoglobin, that contain iron. The word "heme" means "blood" in Greek. If porphyrins are not broken down, they can then begin to accumulate in the skin, where exposure to sunlight activates them and damage to the skin follows. It just so happens that the decrease in quantity and activity of UROD is a result of iron overload.

Iron and the Hypothalamus, Pituitary Gland, and Gonads

Gonads refer to the reproductive organs found in males (testicles) and females (ovaries). The testicles produce sperm and the ovaries eggs, both of which are necessary for procreation. These organs also secrete various sex hormones important for proper development, puberty, fertility, and libido.

> *Testosterone:* the main hormone produced by the testicles, but also produced in the ovaries and adrenal gland. It is responsible for the maturation of male reproductive organs, muscle growth, voice changes, body hair, and sexual desire.

In females, it plays a role in the functioning of the ovaries as well as helping to keep bones strong.

Estrogen: a female sex hormone that is secreted by the ovaries. Contributes to breast development, accumulation of fat around the thighs and hips, menstrual cycle regulation, and fertility.

Progesterone: another ovarian female sex hormone that plays a role in pregnancy by causing changes in the uterus.

In some cases, iron can accumulate in the testicles themselves, causing them to become underactive and produce inadequate testosterone. However, in hemochromatosis it is more common for the gonads to be impacted by a chain reaction involving the hypothalamus and pituitary gland. The hypothalamus is an area of the brain that makes hormones that regulate body temperature, appetite, thirst, sleep, desire for sex, emotional changes, heart rate, and the release of other hormones from different glands. One such gland is the pituitary gland. From the hypothalamus, gonadotropin-releasing hormone (GnRH) causes the pituitary gland to release hormones such as luteinizing hormone (LH) and follicle-stimulating hormone (FSH), which then stimulate the ovaries and testes.

When the hypothalamus and/or the pituitary gland are affected by iron overload, the condition is known as hypogonadotropic hypogonadism. In this condition there is an absence or insufficiency of the GnRH, LH, and FSH hormones, leading to failure of the gonads. Symptoms include erectile dysfunction, impotence, diminished libido, amenorrhea, and infertility. Generally, females with hemochromatosis develop hypogonadism one to two decades later than males and with less frequency than their male counterparts.

Iron and the Joints

A common and early symptom of iron overload is joint pain. Several studies have interestingly pinpointed that arthropathy (joint disease) in hemochromatosis patients often affects specific sites such as the ankle and joints, or knuckles, of the index and middle fingers. Arthropathy in the knuckles limits their range of motion, which sometimes causes the hand to form into an "iron salute."

A lot is still uncertain about the connection between iron overload and joint pain. Hemochromatosis-related arthropathy has long been considered to be noninflammatory in nature, but a 2017 study conducted in Austria observed otherwise. This study, with the help of ultrasonography, looked at individuals with hemochromatosis who had arthropathy, those with hemochromatosis but without the arthropathy, and those with hand osteoarthritis (degenerative joint disease). The collected data showed that there was a high prevalence of inflammation in those with arthropathy, similar to those with osteoarthritis.

It is also believed that individuals with hemochromatosis who develop osteoarthritis may be experiencing a buildup of iron in the synovium and cartilage (both are tissues that line the surface of joints) along with accumulation of ferritin in the synovial fluid.

It appears that once joint problems arise, treatment for hemochromatosis might not be effective for all in alleviating joint discomfort. Improvement has been reported in upward of 30% of patients. Another approach—to address the resulting inflammation—has been seen to offer relief. Some individuals require operations to address the problem. Of course, early detection and treatment of hemochromatosis itself is the best-case scenario in the prevention of severe injury to the joints.

Chapter 3

Screening and Diagnosing

With so much on the line for individuals with hereditary hemo-chromatosis, it may seem like a wonder that measures to screen the general public have not been taken. Several organizations such as the US Preventive Services Task Force and the Centers for Disease Control and Prevention (CDC) do not support routine screening without any signs or symptoms, unless there is a family history of someone affected by the disorder. One rationale is that it would be like opening a can of worms with potentially large numbers of people with the mutated HFE gene who might never actually have the clinical disease pursuing uncalled-for exams and treatments. Instead, organizations such as the American Association for the Study of Liver Diseases (AASLD) recommend that individuals be screened if they (a) are a first-degree relative of someone with hereditary hemochromatosis or (b) experience symptoms. Children should only be screened if they have one parent with hemochromatosis and the other parent is found to have the genetic mutation. The AASLD also recommends that individuals with abnormal iron laboratory studies or liver disease be evaluated for hemochromatosis.

Blood Testing

To screen for the presence of hereditary hemochromatosis, a blood test is often the first step taken to establish iron levels in the body. Genetic testing can confirm a genetic mutation but will not shed light on the state of iron metabolism. For this reason, there are several blood tests in particular that are administered to detect iron overload and screen for hemochromatosis.

Serum Iron (SI): measures how much iron is in the blood. Typically elevated in individuals with hemochromatosis.

Serum Ferritin (SF): measures how much iron is stored in the body. Certain disorders other than hemochromatosis, such as rheumatoid arthritis as well as infections, inflammation, and some medications, are also known to increase ferritin levels. Evaluating SF in conjunction with SI and transferrin saturation (TS) is more meaningful in relation to iron overload in those with hemochromatosis. It is unreliable on its own.

Total Iron Binding Capacity (TIBC): measures how much transferrin, iron's transport mechanism, is available to bind iron. Low levels of TIBC mean that there is not much transferrin available to bind to iron and carry it along. This suggests iron overload.

Transferrin Saturation (TS): measures how much of the transferrin protein is saturated with iron. Measured as a percentage, it is calculated by dividing the SI by the TIBC and multiplying by 100. Able to detect hemochromatosis early on as it is one of the first lab markers to change.

Genetic Testing

If the blood test suggests that there could be hemochromatosis, the diagnosis can then be confirmed with a genetic test. The genetic test can be carried out using a blood or saliva sample, or even just a cheek swab. This test typically screens for some of the more common genetic mutations associated with hemochromatosis, such as C282Y, H63D, and S65C. In recent years, it's become possible to test for some of the more uncommon mutations as well.

Liver Biopsy

On occasion, additional measures are necessary to confirm the diagnosis and to determine the degree of iron accumulation in organs. One such measure, the liver biopsy, is recommended for individuals who are diagnosed with hereditary hemochromatosis and also show elevated liver enzymes or serum ferritin levels greater than 1,000 nanograms per milliliter (ng/mL). These markers suggest the presence of liver disease. A liver biopsy can then further pinpoint how much iron has deposited in the liver, the degree of scar tissue formation, or even cancer.

Since liver biopsy is an invasive procedure with slight risk of complications, researchers have found other methods that can often be used in place of the biopsy procedure. Magnetic resonance imaging (MRI) is a noninvasive and highly sensitive method of detecting iron in the liver. The other upside of utilizing the MRI is that it can also be used to evaluate the state of other organs, such as the heart.

Phlebotomy

Iron overload can also be assessed through quantitative phlebotomy. This procedure is used on individuals who do not require or are not good candidates for a liver biopsy. This technique involves drawing blood and then calculating how much iron has been removed. When iron depletion is achieved after the removal of at least 4 grams of mobilizable iron, the individual is considered to have iron overload.

Chapter 4

Treatment

Therapeutic Phlebotomy

The most widely accepted method for de-ironing (removal of excess Iron) is a procedure known as therapeutic phlebotomy (sometimes referred to as blood-letting or venesection). This tech nique removes blood and is carried out in the same way a typical blood donation would be. Unlike donating blood, however, a thera- peutic phlebotomy needs to be prescribed. At present, phlebotomy is seen as the gold standard because it has withstood the test of time and has a reputation as effective, safe, widely available, and inexpensive.

The frequency of treatments and the amount of blood removed is dependent on the severity of iron overload as well as the person's age, gender, build, overall health, and tolerance. In the beginning, treatment may be more aggressive in order to quickly reach normal levels. According to the AASLD, the goal is to achieve a ferritin level between 50 and 100 ng/mL; however, the Iron Disorders Institute defines the ideal range as 50 to 150 ng/mL (with 50 to 75 ng/mL being the range when therapy is first initiated). To meet this goal, a unit (roughly 1 pint) of blood per week is typically removed. With every unit, ferritin levels decrease by approximately 30 ng/mL. This could mean that upward of 50 phlebotomy treatments may be necessary to achieve a normal level. Afterward, the patient enters a maintenance phase to prevent iron from veering outside an acceptable range. During this phase, phlebotomies are performed less frequently.

A noticeable improvement in energy levels and skin pigmentation often follows treatment with therapeutic phlebotomy. Another benefit can include the reversal of most ailments that developed in response to an overload in iron, especially if the condition was in an early stage. This is why it is so important to diagnose and manage hemochromatosis early on. In addition to decreasing their risk of morbidity and mortality, individuals who undergo therapeutic phlebotomy are often able to help others by donating their blood to those in need of blood transfusions. This may be surprising but, remember, hemochromatosis is not a transmittable disorder, and the amount of iron in a unit of blood from someone with hemo-chromatosis is no different than that of the average donor (the excess iron is stored in the organs). In 1999, the Food and Drug Administration recognized the blood from individuals with hemo-chromatosis to be a safe product for transfusion.

Apheresis

Another treatment method that has shown promise is apheresis. In its most recent guidelines, the American Society for Apheresis (ASFA) noted this procedure to be a satisfactory form of therapy for hereditary hemochromatosis. This alternative approach does not remove whole blood like the phlebotomy but rather extracts the red blood cells (which contain iron) and returns the remaining blood components to the patient. It also appears to be a more efficient method due to its ability to remove nearly 1,000 ml of red blood cells in a single treatment. Therapeutic phlebotomy only manages to remove approximately 250 ml of red blood cells at a time.

Some studies have found that by being more efficient, apheresis allows individuals who undergo the process to get away with fewer treatments and more time between sessions. One study even found that apheresis is no more expensive than therapeutic phlebotomy. However, another study published in 2014 did not find apheresis to be more effectual or comparable in cost to phlebotomy. Rather, it observed that despite apheresis being able to rapidly reduce ferritin levels at the start and decrease the number of procedures each patient requires, individuals take just as long to reach the recommended ferritin levels. It also found it to be more expensive and less widely available than phlebotomy treatments.

Iron Chelation Therapy

Iron chelation therapy is another avenue sometimes taken, typically when phlebotomy cannot be performed. Chelation therapy involves taking drugs such as deferoxamine, deferasirox, or deferiprone to bind to iron and carry it out of the body. Some can be taken orally while others, like deferoxamine, are most effective when infused into the veins or under the skin. Because these agents are not as efficient as phlebotomy, are costly, and are often accompanied by many side effects like stomach aches, nausea, vomiting, diarrhea, and, in some cases, loss of sight or hearing, they are utilized when other methods are contraindicated.

Chapter 5

Sources of Iron

By now it should be clear that too much iron is poisonous to the body. It can overburden nearly every organ, leading to disease and premature death. On the opposite end of the spectrum, a deficiency of iron carries its own set of problems, with complications ranging from depression to cognitive delays in children. So, what is this vital micronutrient that the body can sometimes struggle to live with but certainly cannot live without?

Iron is a mineral that the human body does not make on its own but can absorb from the consumption of certain plant and animal products. Dietary iron comes in two forms: heme and nonheme. Animal products like meat, fish, and poultry are rich sources of heme iron. Plant-based foods like fruits, vegetables, enriched grains, tofu, fortified cereals, and nuts mostly consist of the nonheme version of iron. Compared to heme iron, which has an absorption rate of 15% to 35%, nonheme iron has a lower absorption rate of 2% to 20%. The rate of absorption differs due to heme iron being able to move through the intestinal wall while nonheme iron needs to go through a series of steps before it can be absorbed. The form of iron in nonheme iron is ferric iron. Humans are unable to absorb ferric iron. It first needs to link to oxygen to convert to ferric oxide. This form then has to combine with hydrochloric acid (the acid inside the stomach) to become ferrous iron, which is the form that the body is able to absorb.

When heme iron is available in conjunction with nonheme iron, the absorption rate of the nonheme iron increases. For example, pairing lamb chops with broccoli will promote the absorption of the iron in the broccoli. Of course, individuals with hemochromatosis have a much more exaggerated rate of absorption. There are, however, various measures that can be taken to inhibit or enhance the absorption of iron. Also, certain iron-rich foods contain other components that get in the way of iron absorption (more on this in Chapter 7). Understanding the distinction between the different forms of iron and what influences their bioavailability is helpful in managing hemochromatosis from a dietary standpoint.

Iron-Rich Animal-Based Foods	Iron-Rich Plant-Based Foods
Beef	Almonds
Chicken	Beans
Clams	Brazil nuts
Fish	Broccoli
Lamb	Dried apricots
Liver	Dried figs
Mussels	Green leafy vegetables
Oysters	Hazelnuts
Pork	Iron-fortified cereals
Shrimp	Lentils
Turkey	Molasses
Veal	Peanut butter
Venison	Sesame seeds
	Sunflower seeds
	Tofu

Dried fruit has a higher concentration of iron because most of its water has been removed.

Certain types of foods can vary widely even if they are within the same category. Take cereal, for example. General Mills Total provides 18 mg of iron in a single serving. Meanwhile, General Mills Fiber One offers 4.5 mg of iron in a single serving. Both are iron-fortified but to varying degrees. To help you determine the amount of iron in a product that is packaged or canned, make sure to review the nutrition facts label.

All of the information noted on a nutrition facts label pertains to the serving size of that particular product. If the serving size is ½ cup and you consume 1 cup, then you are getting double the amount of iron noted on the label. To help you evaluate the amount of iron in a serving, the percent daily value is the next place to look. As a rule of thumb, 5 percent or less is considered to be low and 20% or more is high.

The percent daily value when at 100% translates to 18 mg of iron. If a serving has 10% iron, then that food contains 1.8 mg of iron. Generally, 100% daily value is how much an adult needs in a single day based on a 2,000-calorie diet. Certain foods offer 100% of the daily value in a single serving! Such is the case with General Mills Total cereal. So make sure to do your due diligence, and read the label.

Chapter 6

Lifestyle Modification

While hereditary hemochromatosis isn't something that can be brought on to oneself, there are certain lifestyle habits that can either expedite the progression of the disease or help manage it better.

Alcohol

Alcohol consumption is stitched into the fabric of social interaction. It is how we celebrate and how we unwind. Public perception, shaped by various studies, is that moderate alcohol consumption can be protective against diseases like dementia and heart disease. Yet, to this day, the evidence is complicated, as there is some support surrounding potential benefits to moderate amounts of alcohol, but a recent study concluded that no amount of alcohol is beneficial. Interpretation of all of the available data leaves experts certain of only two things: further research is warranted, and alcohol is not necessary for well-being and longevity.

When hereditary hemochromatosis is in the picture, the stance on alcohol becomes a bit more concrete. Alcohol increases iron stores. It is also mostly metabolized in the liver. Just like excess iron, alcohol causes oxidative stress and injury. In the presence of an iron overload condition, the addition of alcohol can only magnify and speed up the deleterious effects to the liver.

Dietary recommendations:

- Undoubtedly, those with hereditary hemochromatosis should avoid excessive intake of alcohol at all costs or else significantly increase the risk of cirrhosis and liver cancer at a younger age.

- Even moderate drinking, defined as two drinks per day for men and one drink per day for women, is discouraged.

Supplements

In general, supplementing with iron is only recommended in instances where there is an iron deficiency or a risk of deficiency. In the presence of an iron-overload condition, it is ill-advised. The other consideration is vitamin C (ascorbic acid) since it aids in the absorption of iron. If selecting a multivitamin, it is important to ensure that the formulation is free of both iron and vitamin C.

Vitamin C in the Diet

Even though vitamin C enhances the absorption of iron, it is not necessary to limit intake of vitamin C–rich foods like fruits and vegetables. First, these foods are incredibly nutritious and are a great source of vitamins, minerals, antioxidants, and fiber. Second, ascorbic acid can only accelerate the absorption of iron when consumed at the same time as foods that contain iron. With a savvy approach to meal planning (see the Two-Week Meal Plan on page 46), it is possible to enjoy all of the benefits of vitamin C–rich foods without contributing to iron overload. More on vitamin C on page 33.

Smoking

Most would agree that smoking does the body way more harm than good. It has been linked to impaired hearing, macular degeneration, cancer, heart disease, emphysema, increased risk of diabetes, erectile dysfunction, and a weakened immune system. As with hemochromatosis, it can negatively impact practically every organ in the body. Furthermore, smoking has been noted to increase iron stores. One study found an interplay between smoking and alcohol consumption, where those who smoked a lot and had a moderate intake of alcohol were susceptible to elevated iron stores. Those who drank a lot, however, were more inclined to have excess iron whether they once smoked or smoked fewer than 10 cigarettes per day. Another study observed that women who smoked during their pregnancy had greater ferritin levels than those who were nonsmokers. Those who smoked heavily and had chronic hepatitis C were found to also have increased levels of iron. With all of this in mind, taking measures to quit smoking is recommended.

Raw Shellfish

If you happen to enjoy raw oysters and have been thinking of cutting back due to their high iron content, another factor might sway you to avoid them entirely. Raw shellfish are susceptible to having *Vibrio vulnificus*, a species of bacteria that thrives in warm seawater. For the average person, ingestion of this bacteria may mean an unpleasant bout of foodborne illness. With hemochromatosis in the equation, such an infection could be life-threatening since the combination of liver disease or a suppressed immune system and the tendency of *V. vulnificus* to blossom in an iron-rich environment may result in sepsis (the body's response to an infection that can quickly escalate to tissue damage, organ failure, and death). In fact, this combination happens to be lethal in 50% of cases.

Iron-Fortified and Iron-Enriched Foods

Iron-fortified breakfast cereals and iron-enriched breads are commonly found in supermarkets nationwide. The popular practice of iron fortification is intended to prevent iron deficiency in the general population, as this is a widespread problem. Since overload rather than deficiency is the concern for someone with hemochromatosis, the question is then, should these foods be avoided?

One point to consider is the quantity of such products in the diet, since intake can easily go beyond the recommended daily allowance. Another factor is the *form* of iron being used in the product because not all iron compounds are created equal. They are all nonheme versions but differ in their degree of bioavailability. The iron fortifiers that are the most efficiently absorbed are NaFeEDTA and ferrous bisglycinate. These additives, particularly ferrous bis-glycinate, are highly bioavailable even in the presence of certain iron inhibitors. It is best to avoid any products that contain them. Ferrous sulfate, on the other hand, has a fairly low bioavailability.

One study carried out on a small group of men with hemochromatosis found that consuming a diet with iron-fortified products caused a 12% increase in their iron uptake. Meanwhile, a diet lacking iron-fortified products allowed for a reduction in the number of phlebotomies necessary during the maintenance phase.

Dietary recommendations:

- When possible, avoid iron-fortified and iron-enriched products.
- If consuming foods that have been fortified with iron, ensure that they do not have the NaFeEDTA or ferrous bisglycinate version, enjoy sparingly, and have them in a meal that also includes an iron inhibitor (see Chapter 7 for more on iron inhibitors).

Cast-Iron and Stainless-Steel Cookware

Nonheme iron can also find its way into the foods you eat from kitchen equipment that you use. Anything made of stainless steel contains various metals, one of which is iron. Another source is cast-iron cookware. Both of these materials leach iron into the foods being cooked, particularly those that are cooked longer and include acidic ingredients such as tomato sauce or vinegar. With so many cookware options on the market, it's best to avoid cooking with stainless-steel or cast-iron pots and pans.

Chapter 7

Dietary Enhancers and Inhibitors of Iron Absorption

Various dietary substances have been seen to either inhibit or enhance the absorption of iron. While it may be tempting to immediately decide to avoid any and all enhancers, this is not recommended. As you make your way through this chapter, you will see that many enhancers still have an important place in a well-rounded diet. They are often found in foods that contribute many health benefits, so it would actually be a great disservice to overall wellness to avoid them. Instead, take note of where they could fit into your diet best so that you get the best of both worlds!

Dietary Enhancers of Iron Absorption

Vitamin C

Vitamin C (ascorbic acid) is a nutrient that the body needs but cannot make it on its own. Benefits span antioxidant properties, collagen production, and the support of a healthy immune system. This translates to helping keep blood vessels, teeth, gums, and bones healthy. It also means that this nutrient plays a part in wound healing, keeping skin smooth and youthful, and helping the body overcome a cold faster. One of vitamin C's other qualities is its ability to increase the absorption of iron.

All vegetables and fruits contain some amount of vitamin C, with certain ones being better sources than others. Here are some of the top natural sources of this nutrient:

VEGETABLES	FRUITS
Asparagus	Avocados
Bell peppers	Blackberries
Bitter melon	Blueberries
Bok choy	Cantaloupes
Broccoli	Grapefruits
Broccoli rabe	Guavas
Brussels sprouts	Kiwis
Cabbage	Lychees
Cauliflower	Mandarins
Collard greens	Mangoes
Kale	Oranges
Kohlrabi	Papayas
Potatoes	Persimmons
Snow peas	Pineapples
Sweet potatoes	Raspberries
Tomatoes	Strawberries
Turnip greens	Tangerines

Certain dietary components, such as calcium, inhibit iron absorption, but ascorbic acid is actually powerful enough to still increase the absorption of iron even in their presence. Prolonged storage and cooking damage vitamin C and lessen its ability to increase iron absorption. Also, vitamin C has an opportunity to enhance the absorption of iron only if consumed in the same meal as the iron-containing foods. Since vitamin C offers so many health benefits and is commonly found in produce that offers additional health-promoting compounds, like antioxidants, fiber, and minerals, it is important to maintain these foods in a daily diet.

Dietary recommendations:

- When eating a meal with iron-rich ingredients, such as meat, rather than eliminate vegetables high in vitamin C, consider pairing these foods with cooked vegetables rather than fresh.
- Enjoy vitamin C–rich fruits as a snack, apart from meals with iron-containing foods.

Beta-Carotene

Beta-carotene is a naturally occurring pigment that gives certain fruits and vegetables a vibrant yellow and orange color; think carrots and sweet potatoes. Spinach is also an excellent source of beta-carotene, but is green due to the chlorophyll within the leaves hiding the orange-yellow pigment. Other examples of green-hued foods that are good sources of beta-carotene are collards, kale, turnip greens, and dandelion greens. It is known as a provitamin because the body is able to convert it into vitamin A (retinol). Large amounts of vitamin A can be harmful, but the body will only create as much vitamin A from beta-carotene as it needs, so this is not something to be concerned about. This provitamin is an antioxidant, helping to protect against free radical damage. Studies looking at this provitamin's role in cancer have been mixed, and it appears that any existing protective benefit is probably small. Other studies have suggested that beta-carotene may play a role in protecting against heart disease. While its role in disease prevention is not entirely clear, it is undoubtedly beneficial for its ability to create vitamin A safely with no risk of overdose. Vitamin A supports eyesight and proper functioning of organs, the reproductive system, and the immune system.

Beta-carotene has been noted to increase iron absorption, even in the presence of iron inhibitors.

Dietary recommendations:

- Similar to the case of vitamin C, since beta-carotene is found in nutrient-packed fruits and vegetables, it is not necessary to eliminate food sources of this provitamin.

Fructose

When thinking about sugar, most people envision white, crystal-like granules that are added for sweetness to many of the foods and beverages that we consume. While accurate, this only describes one type of sugar by the name of sucrose. Meanwhile, our food supply also has a variety of other naturally occurring sugars, like lactose, maltose, galactose, and so on. Since the 1960s, researchers have attempted to decipher if certain sugars are able to influence the absorption of nonheme iron. Although this area would benefit from further research, several studies have singled out one particular type of sugar, fructose. Fructose is found as a simple sugar in fruits and honey, chemically joined to glucose to create sucrose (table sugar), or in a mixture with glucose commonly known as high-fructose corn syrup (HFCS).

One study found that fructose and HFCS enhance iron bioavailability in both the gut and the liver. Since fruit is a source of fructose, it may seem that restriction would be necessary, but other studies don't necessarily point in that direction. Researchers examining the impact of non-citrus fruits on iron levels in individuals with hereditary hemochromatosis did not observe an increase in iron stores. This could be due to the fruits containing certain iron inhibitors alongside the fructose, counteracting any effect that it alone would have. On the contrary, the Framingham Heart Study found fruit to enhance iron absorption. This study differed in that it included citrus fruits, a good source of vitamin C, which is a known enhancer of iron absorption.

Dietary recommendations:

- Avoid products with high-fructose corn syrup, like sodas, candies, and condiments.
- Aim to have around 1½ to 2 cups of fruit per day, consuming vitamin C–rich fruits apart from meals containing iron. Since heat destroys vitamin C, having cooked fruit is another great option.

Meat, Fish, and Poultry

Meat, fish, and poultry are good sources of the better-absorbed heme iron but also contain an MFP factor (MFP stands for meat, fish, and poultry and precisely what these factors are have yet to be clearly pinpointed), which increases the absorption of non-heme iron. Several studies have observed an enhancing effect in the absorption of nonheme iron, particularly in meals consisting of cereal or beans, with the inclusion of these animal products. This MFP factor only influences the absorption of nonheme iron that is a part of the same meal and does not have a lingering effect that can impact the absorption of nonheme iron in foods eaten at a later time. For example, when eating a meat and bean chili, the heme iron housed in the meat will be well absorbed and due to the MFP factor, the nonheme iron in the beans will be better absorbed than usual. To put it in perspective, one study calculated that 1 gram of meat, fish, or poultry had an enhancing effect comparable to that of 1 milligram of ascorbic acid (vitamin C).

Dietary recommendations:

- Enjoy well-balanced, vegetarian meals on occasion to benefit from the various nutrients and minerals without enhancing the absorption of iron.
- Consider joining the Meatless Monday movement, a campaign established in association with the Johns Hopkins Bloomberg School of Public Health. Focusing more on fruits, vegetables, legumes, whole grains, and dairy products once a week is not just an opportunity to limit iron absorption but also a chance to cut down on intake of saturated fats and reduce your carbon footprint!

Dietary Inhibitors of Iron Absorption

Curcumin

Curcumin, a key phytochemical nestled within a spice called turmeric, is often touted for its health benefits. It holds anti-inflammatory and antioxidant properties, with some evidence to suggest that it also possesses anticancer abilities. Since many health conditions are associated with oxidative stress and inflammation, it is not surprising to see curcumin make a positive impact on a long list of diseases. Studies have shown curcumin to help alleviate pain in osteoarthritis, manage anxiety, improve choles- terol levels, and better manage metabolic syndrome by enhancing insulin sensitivity, decreasing blood pressure, and reducing fat gain.

While curcumin has many potential health benefits, its bioavailabil- ity is poor as it does not easily absorb in the body and is also quickly metabolized and eliminated. For this reason, most research studies do not just look at curcumin alone but include agents that enhance the bioavailability of this chemical. A popular additive is piperine, which is found in black pepper. According to "Curcumin: A Review of Its Effects on Human Health," it can increase the bioavailability of curcumin by 2,000%.

Curcumin also happens to be similar in structure to beta-caro- tene with one study noting it to increase the bioaccessibility of iron in food grains. However, the amount at which this effect was observed was much larger than the typical amount of turmeric an average person would use in a dish. On the other hand, studies carried out on rodents found curcumin to have an iron-chelating effect, meaning that it was able to reduce iron in their bodies. One study, for example, observed rats overloaded with iron to experi- ence a reduction in iron in the liver and spleen following exposure to curcumin.

Dietary recommendations:

- While animal studies do not always accurately predict a reaction in humans, it is still beneficial to include a spice like turmeric in cooking for its antioxidant properties.

Polyphenols

Polyphenols are a group of various antioxidants that naturally occur in plant-based products. Sources include fruits, vegetables, cocoa, herbs, tea, coffee, and red wine. During the digestive process these antioxidants are released from foods and beverages and link to iron. This newly formed complex gets in the way of the iron being absorbed.

Tannins

One type of polyphenol known as tannins is found in plant substances that can be quite astringent and bitter in taste. Unripe fruits and concentrated teas are good examples of that unique mouthfeel attributed to the presence of tannins. Tannins have the tendency to accumulate in fruit peels and the bran of grains. For instance, peeled apples will not have as many tannins as apples with the peel. Overall, they are found in most plant-based foods. Some common food sources are grains (barley and sorghum), beverages (tea, wine, and coffee), chocolate (cacao beans, chocolate liquor, and cocoa powder), fruits (apples, berries, cherries, cranberries, grapes, and pomegranates), legumes (beans, chickpeas, black-eyed peas, and lentils), nuts (cashews, peanuts, pecans, and walnuts), and vegetables (squash and rhubarb).

Tannins have been known to bind to nonheme iron in the gut, inhibiting its absorption. Research focusing on individuals with hemochromatosis has mostly evaluated tea intake and has paved the way to a common recommendation of enjoying black tea with meals to cut down on the amount of iron absorbed. "The Impact of Tannin Consumption on Iron Bioavailability and Status," a review article that looked at 37 different studies, found that while intake of tannins did reduce the bioavailability of iron, this effect was not always observed when a diet high in tannins was consumed over a long period of time, suggesting that the body can adapt.

While tannins may play a role in lowering the absorption of nonheme iron, it is best to steer clear of high concentrations, particularly if liver damage is in the picture. It is best to stay away from certain herbs that have been seen to be harmful to the liver due to their tannin concentrations. Examples of such herbs are American cranesbill, bayberry, bilberry, blue flag, buckthorn, kola nut, cowslip, damiana, lady's mantle, locust bean, oak, and poplar. These herbs also go by many other names, making it important to do thorough research and to consult with a doctor prior to taking any herbal supplements.

Dietary recommendations:

- It is not necessary to overly emphasize the consumption of tannin-rich products. Instead, strategize to include a tannin-containing food or beverage with a meal to potentially decrease the amount of nonheme iron that would get absorbed. For instance, rather than sipping a mug of black tea between meals, enjoy it with your meal.

Chlorogenic Acid

Another type of polyphenol that has an inhibitory effect on iron is chlorogenic acid. Coffee is one of the richest dietary sources of chlorogenic acid and, based on consumption trends in the United States, it happens to be a major source of this polyphenol. Roughly 80% of adults in the US drink coffee, with 60% consuming coffee every day. A single cup of coffee can decrease iron absorption by approximately 60%. One study focused on an elderly population in the Framingham Heart Study found the consumption of one cup of coffee a week helped lower ferritin levels by 1%. Coffee's effect on iron absorption, of course, can also be attributed to its other substances, such as the tannins described on page 39.

Dietary recommendations:

- Coffee lovers, rejoice! This popular beverage joins the ranks of tea in its ability to inhibit the absorption of iron and can be enjoyed with a meal.

Oxalates

Oxalates are substances that come from oxalic acid, which is found in many plant foods in varying concentrations. Examples of foods with high levels of oxalate are spinach, rhubarb, and Swiss chard. Oxalates have been known to have an inhibitory effect on certain minerals, yet it's not entirely clear whether iron is one of them. The literature has observed oxalate-rich foods to reduce iron absorption; however, whether the oxalates deserve the credit is not so certain.

A 2006 study conducted in India looked at the bioavailability of iron in leafy green vegetables and found oxalic acid plays a role in inhibiting iron absorption. The researchers observed oxalic acid, tannin, and phytic acid to inhibit iron absorption, with the oxalic acid being the largest factor for the decrease. Another, very small study from 2007 that took place in Switzerland suggests that oxalic acid does not play a role in the inhibition of iron absorption and that any inhibitory factor on iron found in spinach cannot be attributed to oxalic acid but rather to the presence of other inhibitors. Meanwhile, another study carried out in 2005 found that although leafy green vegetables like spinach have a low bioavailability of iron in a raw state, when cooked the iron becomes significantly more available, and this may be due to a decrease in oxalic acid. When boiled, spinach loses upward of 87% of its oxalate content and iron availability improves. However, it is also worth noting that cooking results in a decrease of other anti-nutrients (naturally found substances that get in the way of the absorption of certain nutrients) like phytic acid and polyphenols.

Dietary recommendations:

- Whether it is the oxalic acid or the action of another anti-nutrient that is responsible for the low availability of iron in spinach, the takeaway here is do not be fearful of including raw spinach in your diet. Iron levels increase when spinach is cooked or prepared with iron enhancers like vitamin C–rich products.

Phytic Acid

The standard American diet (SAD) is characterized by an emphasis on saturated fats, animal proteins, salt, and sugar. It paints a picture of overconsumption of processed foods and inadequate intake of fiber-rich produce, grains, and healthy fats. Besides being high in calories and low in nutritional value, the SAD way of eating is low in a particular compound that is quite valuable to someone dealing with hemochromatosis—phytic acid.

Phytic acid is the storage form of phosphorus. Found primarily in unprocessed plant foods, it can bind to minerals like iron-forming phytates. This compound is commonly found in whole grains, legumes, seeds, and nuts. Some examples of foods high in phytic acid include wheat bran/germ, soybeans/soy concentrate, sesame seeds, almonds, walnuts, Brazil nuts, and kidney beans.

When phytic acid is bound to iron, the body's ability to absorb the iron is reduced, causing it to get excreted out of the body. In addition to inhibiting the absorption of iron, phytic acid has been associated with the prevention of cancer, diabetes, cardiovascular disease, and kidney stones. Talk about a win-win!

Dietary recommendations:

- Although many phytate-rich foods are often high in iron, this iron is not well-absorbed because of the phytates. Continue to incorporate them into your diet.

Eggs

Even though eggs contain a decent amount of iron, they are still an egg-cellent choice for someone with hemochromatosis. While the yolk houses iron, it also contains a phosphoprotein (a protein that contains phosphorus) known as phosvitin, which binds to most of the iron, creating a phosvitin-iron complex. Under such conditions, the bioavailability of iron is reduced. One study looking at Danish men with the HFE gene found eggs did not alter iron status, even when more than four eggs were consumed over the span of a week. Another study observed the inclusion of a single egg reduced the absorption of iron in that meal by 28%.

Besides addressing the issue with iron, eggs are a great source of high-quality protein and are full of nutrients like biotin, choline, vitamin A, lutein, zeaxanthin, and vitamin D. These nutrients support healthy bones, the immune system, liver function, and eye health. If you're concerned about the cholesterol content of the yolk, don't be! The 2015–2020 Dietary Guidelines have done away with the recommendation to limit the consumption of dietary cholesterol to 300 mg per day. Meanwhile, the American Heart Association advises that seven eggs a week can be part of a healthy diet.

Dietary recommendations:

- Contrary to popular belief, eggs should remain in the diet.

Calcium

An abundant array of foods are great sources of calcium, like dairy products (ricotta, milk, yogurt, cheese), dark green leafy vegetables (collard greens, turnip greens, kale), canned fish with bones, calcium-fortified tofu, and calcium-fortified milk alternatives (almond milk, rice milk, soy milk). This mineral happens to be very important to overall health and well-being. It is involved in the building and maintenance of strong bones and teeth, transmission of signals through the nerves, secretion of hormones, and contraction of muscles.

The added bonus is that calcium has been seen to inhibit the absorption of iron. One study looking at a Spanish Mediterranean population with an HFE gene mutation found calcium to benefit iron status, particularly in males. Another study involving a large number of Danish blood donors found that those living in areas with a high calcium concentration in the water had lower iron stores and were more susceptible to developing an iron deficiency. According to the National Institutes of Health Office of Dietary Supplements, calcium may have the ability to decrease the bioavailability of heme and nonheme iron.

Dietary recommendations:

- Make calcium-rich foods a consistent part of your daily diet, especially since some, like dairy products, are low in iron themselves and may possibly inhibit the uptake of iron in the meal.

Chapter 8

Recipes

With a little mindfulness, you can be well on your way to a varied and delicious way of eating while cutting back on the amount of iron you absorb. The hemochromatosis-friendly diet is not overly complicated nor very restrictive. Rather, it places greater emphasis on the nonheme version of iron and animal proteins that have lower concentrations of heme iron, while also incorporating various inhibitors as discussed in Chapter 7. To help inhibit iron further, make it a habit to enjoy some tea or coffee with your meals. Decaffeinated coffee contains comparable amounts of antioxidants to regular coffee and is an acceptable choice for the polyphenol benefits.

Prior to the recipes, I've included a Two-Week Meal Plan to get you on the path to a hemochromatosis-friendly diet. Most recipes included here require a limited number of ingredients and are easy to follow, ensuring that no matter your lifestyle or skill set in the kitchen, you will not be intimidated! Judge your serving size according to your specific nutritional needs, using the nutritional information provided with each recipe to help you determine how many servings to have in your meals. Remember, you are also never limited to these recipes—any cuisine can be enjoyed, with just a few tweaks along the way.

Please be advised that everyone's journey with hereditary hemochromatosis is different and depending on your experience, individualized recommendations may be warranted. It is important to consult with your doctor and registered dietitian prior to making any adjustments. For example, while tannins are an inhibitor of iron absorption, large amounts are not suitable if you have liver damage.

TWO-WEEK MEAL PLAN

	WEEK ONE
MONDAY	**BREAKFAST** • Raspberry Truffle Smoothie (page 55)
	SNACK • Brown Rice Pudding (page 122)
	LUNCH • Smoky Lentil Burgers (page 84) • Zucchini Salad (page 78)
	SNACK • Apple • String cheese
	DINNER • Quinoa (Bean-less) Chili, (page 102) • Eggplant Rollups (page 95)
TUESDAY	**BREAKFAST** • Turmeric Latte (page 113) • Breakfast Mocha Quinoa (page 60)
	SNACK • Apple Chips (page 124)
	LUNCH • Leftover Smoky Lentil Burger sandwich • Mixed vegetable salad
	SNACK • Leftover Brown Rice Pudding
	DINNER • Creamy Cod (page 100) • Roasted Vegetable Medley (page 106) • Mashed potato

Living Well with Hemochromatosis

WEDNESDAY	**BREAKFAST** • Iced Chai (page 114) • High-Protein Overnight Oats (page 56)
	SNACK • Leftover Apple Chips
	LUNCH • Shiitake BLT (page 107) • Mixed Leaf Caesar (page 81) • Caesar Dressing (page 82)
	SNACK • Banana Soft Serve (page 125)
	DINNER • Spring Rolls (page 92) with Peanut Sauce (page 94) • Roasted Vegetable Medley (page 106)
THURSDAY	**BREAKFAST** • Iced Chai (page 114) • Swiss Chard Quiche (page 63)
	SNACK • Pineapple • Cottage cheese
	LUNCH • Bean Chili (page 108) • Mixed vegetable salad with avocado
	SNACK • Banana • String cheese
	DINNER • Leftover Spring Rolls with Peanut Sauce • Cheesy Broccoli (page 76)

FRIDAY	**BREAKFAST** • Turmeric Latte (page 113) • Farmer Cheese Pancakes (page 59)
	SNACK • Mojito Fruit Salad Parfait Snack (page 71)
	LUNCH • Vegan Nourish Bowl (page 90) • Green Goddess Dressing (page 91)
	SNACK • Frozen Yogurt Cups (page 118)
	DINNER • Earthy Haddock (page 101) • Leftover Cheesy Broccoli • Brown rice
SATURDAY	**BREAKFAST** • Latte • Green Bean Frittata (page 96) • Whole wheat toast with mashed avocado
	SNACK • Leftover Frozen Yogurt Cups
	LUNCH • Leftover Earthy Haddock • Macaroni Casserole (page 86) • Side salad with leftover Green Goddess Dressing
	SNACK • Celery sticks • Peanut butter
	DINNER • Black Tea Marinated Tofu (page 66) • Wild rice • Asparagus

SUNDAY	BREAKFAST • Turmeric Latte (page 113) • Banana Pancakes (page 58)
	SNACK • Mixed Fruit Kompot (page 77)
	LUNCH • Mushroom Soup (page 88) • Salmon Salad (page 80) • Whole wheat crackers
	SNACK • Tzatziki Toasts (page 72)
	DINNER • Pesto Pasta (page 99) • Leftover Black Tea Marinated Tofu • Roasted Endive (page 75)

WEEK 2	
MONDAY	BREAKFAST • Cappuccino • Lazy Cheese Dumplings (page 69)
	SNACK • Leftover Mixed Fruit Kompot
	LUNCH • Leftover Pesto Pasta • Leftover Black Tea Marinated Tofu
	SNACK • Yogurt • Berries
	DINNER • Leftover Mushroom Soup • Shiitake BLT (page 107)

TUESDAY	**BREAKFAST** • Cappuccino • Buckwheat Porridge (page 61) • Yogurt
	SNACK • Egg Muffins (page 54)
	LUNCH • Caramelized Onion Pizza (page 98) • Mixed vegetable salad
	SNACK • Creamy Fruit Salad Snack (page 70)
	DINNER • Coffee-Rubbed Salmon (page 111) • Polenta Caprese Salad (page 73) • String beans
WEDNESDAY	**BREAKFAST** • Coffee • Leftover Egg Muffins • Whole wheat toast • Yogurt
	SNACK • Leftover Creamy Fruit Salad Snack
	LUNCH • Vegan Nourish Bowl (page 90) • Green Goddess Dressing (page 91)
	SNACK • Walnuts
	DINNER • Leftover Coffee-Rubbed Salmon • Wild rice • Roasted Endive (page 75)

THURSDAY	**BREAKFAST** - Iced latte - Eggs in a Zucchini Nest (page 62)
	SNACK - Poached Pear and Goat Cheese Toast (page 57)
	LUNCH - Kani Salad (page 74) sandwich - Yogurt
	SNACK - Roasted chestnuts
	DINNER - Stroganoff Chicken Meatballs (page 104) - Whole wheat spaghetti - Sautéed cabbage and shredded carrots
FRIDAY	**BREAKFAST** - Raspberry Truffle Smoothie (page 55)
	SNACK - Celery - Peanut butter
	LUNCH - Leftover Stroganoff Chicken Meatballs in a whole wheat pita - Leftover sautéed cabbage and carrots
	SNACK - Brown Rice Pudding (page 122)
	DINNER - Quinoa (Bean-less) Chili (page 102) - Eggplant Rollups (page 95)

SATURDAY	**BREAKFAST** • Iced cappuccino • Eggs with Creamy Polenta (page 64)
	SNACK • Pecans
	LUNCH • Tofu Salad (page 79) sandwich • Vegetable soup
	SNACK • Cottage cheese • Berries
	DINNER • Perfectly Marinated Chicken (page 110) • Stuffed Mushrooms (page 68) • Wild rice
SUNDAY	**BREAKFAST** • Latte • High-Protein Overnight Oats (page 56)
	SNACK • Banana Soft Serve (page 125)
	LUNCH • Tzatziki Toasts (page 72) • Celery and carrot sticks • Yogurt
	SNACK • Leftover Tofu Salad • Whole wheat crackers
	DINNER • Leftover Perfectly Marinated Chicken • Leftover Stuffed Mushrooms • Brown rice

Breakfast

Egg Muffins

Perfect for a grab-and-go breakfast that has some nonheme iron alongside calcium, phosvitin, and polyphenols.

Yield: 12 muffins   **Prep time:** 10 minutes   **Cook time:** 20 minutes

12 large eggs

½ cup low-fat cottage cheese

salt, to taste

black pepper, to taste

1 tablespoon minced fresh basil

12 cherry tomatoes

3 teaspoons grated Parmesan cheese

1. Preheat the oven to 350°F.

2. Lightly spray a muffin tin with nonstick cooking spray, and set aside.

3. Whisk the eggs in a large bowl. Stir in the cottage cheese and basil. Season with salt and pepper, to taste.

4. Pour the mixture into each muffin cup to three-quarters full.

5. Cut each cherry tomato into quarters. Drop four pieces into each muffin cup.

6. Sprinkle the Parmesan evenly over the top of each muffin.

7. Bake for 20 minutes. Allow muffins to cool for a few minutes before removing from pan. Enjoy immediately or freeze and reheat.

Nutrition facts per serving
84 calories | 5.1 g total fat | 1.8 g saturated fat | 1.4 g carbohydrate | 0.2 g fiber | 7.8 g protein | 0.88 mg iron | 43 mg calcium

Raspberry Truffle Smoothie

If you love dark chocolate, then this smoothie is for you! Aside from putting the spotlight on the nonheme form of iron, this smoothie offers plenty of iron inhibitors like calcium, oxalates, and polyphenols in one decadent little package.

Yield: 1 serving   **Prep time:** 5 minutes

1 cup frozen raspberries

1 cup fresh spinach

¾ cup plain Greek yogurt

1 tablespoon cocoa powder

½ frozen banana

½ cup low-fat milk

1 shot espresso

Place all ingredients into a blender and blend until smooth.

Nutrition facts per serving
315 calories | 3 g total fat | 8 g saturated fat | 49.6 g carbohydrate | 13.7 g fiber | 30.1 g protein | 2.43 mg iron | 345 mg calcium

High-Protein Overnight Oats

Yield: 1 serving   **Prep time:** 10 minutes, plus 6 hours to overnight to refrigerate

½ cup low-fat cottage cheese

¼ cup rolled oats

¼ cup nonfat milk

¼ teaspoon ground cinnamon

1 ripe banana, diced into mini cubes

1. Add all ingredients to a bowl, and stir to combine.

2. Pour the mixture into a sealable container, such as a mason jar, cover, and refrigerate overnight or at least 6 hours.

3. Stir and enjoy!

Nutrition facts per serving
305 calories | 3.7 g total fat | 1.4 g saturated fat | 50.8 g carbohydrate | 6.1 g fiber | 20.3 g protein | 1.1 mg iron | 155 mg calcium

Poached Pear and Goat Cheese Toast

Yield: 4 servings   **Prep time:** 10 minutes   **Cook time:** 20 minutes

1 cup water

1 star anise

1 cinnamon stick

¼ teaspoon vanilla extract

1 Bosc pear, peeled, cored, and quartered

4 slices whole wheat bread

4 ounces goat cheese

1. In a small saucepan, combine the water, star anise, cinnamon stick, and vanilla extract, and bring to a boil.

2. Lower heat to medium-low, add pear quarters, and simmer covered for approximately 20 minutes or until tender.

3. Meanwhile, toast the bread.

4. Spread 1 ounce of goat cheese on each slice.

5. Remove the pear from the liquid and thinly slice.

6. Top each goat cheese–covered slice of toast with a quarter of the sliced pear.

Nutrition facts per serving
186 calories | 7.4 g total fat | 4.4 g saturated fat | 21.7 g carbohydrate | 3.7 g fiber | 8.7 g protein | 1.6 mg iron | 68 mg calcium

Banana Pancakes

While iron content appears to be on the higher side, this dish contains phosvitin and a good amount of calcium to help impair the absorption of iron.

Yield: 1 serving (about 10 small pancakes)   **Prep time:** 10 minutes
Cook time: 10 minutes

2 eggs

⅛ teaspoon salt

¼ cup fat-free ricotta cheese

1 ripe banana, mashed with a fork

¼ teaspoon ground cinnamon

1. Whisk the eggs and salt in a medium bowl.

2. Mix in the ricotta cheese, mashed banana, and cinnamon.

3. Preheat a 10-inch skillet over medium heat.

4. Spray the skillet with nonstick cooking spray, and ladle the batter 1 tablespoon at a time into the skillet.

5. Cook for approximately 1 minute until bubbles begin to form on the surface, then flip and cook for another minute or until golden brown. Because ripe bananas are sweet, these pancakes can be enjoyed on their own without any need for syrups or honey.

Nutrition facts per serving
321 calories | 11 g total fat | 3.2 g saturated fat | 37.7 g carbohydrate | 8.2 g fiber | 20.2 g protein | 3.55 mg iron | 326 mg calcium

Farmer Cheese Pancakes

Yield: 4 (5-pancake) servings   **Prep time:** 10 minutes
Cook time: 20 minutes

1 pound farmer cheese	½ cup all-purpose flour
2 eggs	½ teaspoon baking powder
salt, to taste	1 tablespoon olive oil
¼ cup granulated sugar	sour cream, to serve

1. In a large bowl, mix together the farmer cheese, eggs, salt, sugar, flour, and baking powder.

2. Heat the olive oil in a 10-inch skillet over medium heat.

3. Take 1 tablespoon of batter, and with damp hands (to prevent sticking), shape it into a round patty.

4. Place the patty in the skillet and cook until it is golden on each side, about 1 to 2 minutes on each side. Repeat with remaining batter.

5. Serve with sour cream.

Nutrition facts per serving
290 calories | 17 g total fat | 8.1 g saturated fat | 13.5 g carbohydrate | 0 g fiber | 19.5 g protein | 0.52 g iron | 22 mg calcium

Breakfast Mocha Quinoa

Polyphenols, phytates, and calcium make this delicious breakfast an easy pick!

Yield: 2 servings   **Prep time:** 5 minutes   **Cook time:** 30 minutes

½ cup quinoa, rinsed

½ cup unsweetened vanilla almond milk

½ cup strong brewed coffee

pinch of salt

¼ teaspoon vanilla extract

1½ tablespoons semi-sweet chocolate chips

2 teaspoons cocoa powder

4 tablespoons vanilla coconut yogurt, to serve

1. Place the quinoa, almond milk, coffee, salt, vanilla extract, chocolate chips, and cocoa powder into a medium saucepan, and bring to a boil.

2. Once boiling, lower the heat to medium-low and cover with the lid. Allow the quinoa to absorb all of the liquid, about 15 minutes. Turn off the heat and let the quinoa sit covered for another 5 minutes before serving.

3. Spoon the quinoa into bowls and top with 2 tablespoons of vanilla coconut yogurt.

Nutrition facts per serving
247 calories | 7.4 g total fat | 3.2 g saturated fat | 39.7 g carbohydrate | 4.2 g fiber | 7.4 g protein | 2.75 mg iron | 174 mg calcium

Buckwheat Porridge

Yield: 2 servings   **Prep time:** 5 minutes   **Cook time:** 5 minutes

½ cup buckwheat

2 cups low-fat milk

1 teaspoon vanilla extract

1 teaspoon ground cinnamon

1. Cook the buckwheat according to package instructions.

2. In a separate small saucepan, bring the milk, vanilla extract, and cinnamon to a simmer.

3. Pour the liquid over the buckwheat and serve in bowls.

Nutrition facts per serving
206 calories | 3.2 g total fat | 1.5 g saturated fat | 32.4 g carbohydrate | 0.6 g fiber | 11.6 g protein | 0.9 mg iron | 261 mg calcium

Eggs in a Zucchini Nest

Yield: 2 servings   **Prep time:** 5 minutes   **Cook time:** 10 minutes

1 tablespoon olive oil

1 (12-ounce) container zucchini spirals, aka zoodles

salt, to taste

black pepper, to taste

1 cup liquid egg whites (the equivalent of 6 large egg whites)

4 slices whole grain toast

¼ cup shredded reduced-fat mozzarella

chili lime seasoning (optional)

1. Heat the olive oil in a 10-inch pan over medium-high heat. Once hot, sauté the zoodles and season with salt and pepper.

2. Once the zoodles become tender, about 4 minutes, shape them into four nests, leaving an opening in the center for the eggs.

3. Pour ¼ cup egg whites into each nest. Sprinkle the cheese on top of each nest.

4. Cover the pan with a lid for 2 to 4 minutes, or until the egg whites set.

5. Toast the bread in a toaster.

6. Place each nest on a slice of toast.

7. Season with a little more salt and pepper and even a pinch of chili lime seasoning for a little burst of flavor!

Nutrition facts per serving
396 calories | 12 g total fat | 2.2 g saturated fat | 43.5 g carbohydrate | 8 g fiber | 19 g protein | 2.2 mg iron | 100 mg calcium

Swiss Chard Quiche

Yield: 8 servings **Prep time:** 15 minutes **Cook time:** 50 minutes

1 tablespoon avocado oil

2 large leeks, white and pale green portions, sliced

salt, to taste

black pepper, to taste

2½ cups Swiss chard, ribs removed, chopped

1 cup evaporated fat-free milk

5 large eggs

1 teaspoon dried thyme

1 whole wheat pie crust

1. Preheat the oven to 400°F.

2. On the stovetop, heat the avocado oil in a 12-inch pan over medium-high heat and add the leeks, salt, and pepper.

3. Cook the leeks until they soften, about 10 minutes, making sure to stir frequently.

4. Add the Swiss chard and sauté for another 3 minutes, or until the chard is somewhat wilted.

5. While the leek and chard mixture cools, whisk together the milk, eggs, thyme, salt, and pepper in a large bowl.

6. Stir in the Swiss chard and leeks, and pour into the pie crust.

7. Bake the quiche for 20 minutes. Reduce the heat to 350°F and bake for another 15 minutes, or until a knife in the center comes out clean.

8. Allow quiche to cool for 10 minutes before serving.

Nutrition facts per serving
212 calories | 12.8 g total fat | 5.2 g saturated fat | 16.9 g carbohydrate | 2.7 g fiber | 8.5 g protein | 1.57 mg iron | 116 mg calcium

Eggs with Creamy Polenta

Yield: 4 servings   **Prep time:** 5 minutes   **Cook time:** 1 hour

3 cups low-fat milk

2 cups water

1 cup polenta (NOT instant polenta)

salt, to taste

8 eggs, cooked in any style

black pepper, to taste

1. In a medium pot, bring the milk and water to a boil over medium-high heat.

2. Slowly pour in the polenta, whisking the entire time. Continue to stir the mixture until it thickens, about 3 minutes.

3. Lower the heat to medium-low and continue to stir often as the polenta cooks for another 45 minutes, or until it further thickens. If the polenta is too thick, whisk in a little bit of milk. Then season with a little salt to taste.

4. Prepare the eggs in any style.

5. Top each serving of polenta with 2 eggs and season with black pepper to taste.

Nutrition facts per serving
331 calories | 11.9 g total fat | 4.3 g saturated fat | 33.6 g carbohydrate | 2.3 g fiber | 21.2 g protein | 1.75 mg iron | 272 mg calcium

Appetizers and Salads

Black Tea Marinated Tofu

Perfect for sandwiches, the marinated tofu's calcium and poly-phenols will help keep iron absorption down.

Yield: 4 servings   **Prep time:** 20 minutes, plus 90 minutes to overnight to marinate   **Cook time:** 25 minutes

14 ounces extra-firm tofu

2 tea bags black tea

8 ounces boiling water

2 tablespoons reduced-sodium soy sauce

1 teaspoon ground ginger

3 cloves garlic, minced

⅛ teaspoon cayenne pepper

1 tablespoon apple cider vinegar

1. Sandwich the tofu block between two plates and place something heavy on top, like textbooks, and leave for 12 minutes. Use a tofu press if available.

2. In a mug or heat-tolerant measuring cup, steep the tea bags in the hot water for 5 minutes.

3. Discard the water released from the tofu, and slice the tofu into 12 pieces.

4. Once the tea has finished steeping, throw away the tea bags and prepare the marinade in the mug or measuring cup. Mix the soy sauce, ground ginger, garlic, cayenne pepper, and apple cider vinegar into the brewed tea.

5. Lay the tofu slices in a 3-quart glass baking dish, and cover with the marinade. Marinate for at least 90 minutes to overnight in the refrigerator. The longer the tofu sits, the better.

6. Preheat the oven to 400°F. Line a baking sheet with parchment paper and lightly oil. Place the tofu pieces onto the baking sheet.

7. Bake for 25 minutes or until nicely browned.

Nutrition facts per serving
108 calories | 4.7 g total fat | 0.6 g saturated fat | 4.3 g carbohydrate | 1.4 g fiber | 10.1 g protein | 1.87 mg iron | 178 mg calcium

Stuffed Mushrooms

Yield: 4 servings   **Prep time:** 15 minutes   **Cook time:** 15 minutes

12 large white mushrooms, stems removed

2 tablespoons olive oil, divided

salt, to taste

black pepper, to taste

1 onion, chopped

2 cloves garlic, minced

3 tablespoons bread crumbs

3 ounces goat cheese, cut into 12 pieces

2 tablespoons finely chopped fresh parsley

1. Preheat the oven to 400°F.

2. In a large bowl, toss the mushrooms with 1 tablespoon of olive oil, salt, and pepper.

3. Place the mushrooms hole side down on a parchment paper–lined baking sheet and roast for 7 to 8 minutes.

4. In a 10-inch skillet, heat the remaining oil, and sauté the onion and garlic until the onion becomes translucent.

5. Add the bread crumbs to the onion and garlic mixture and season with salt and pepper.

6. Once the mushrooms have cooled for about 10 minutes, place a piece of goat cheese into each mushroom and top with the bread crumb mixture.

7. Bake the mushrooms another 3 minutes, until the bread crumbs are lightly browned.

8. Sprinkle a little parsley over each mushroom and serve.

Nutrition facts per serving
166 calories | 11.3 g total fat | 4 g saturated fat | 10.7 g carbohydrate | 0.8 g fiber | 8.1 g protein | 1 mg iron | 42 mg calcium

Lazy Cheese Dumplings

Yield: 4 servings   **Prep time:** 20 minutes   **Cook time:** 7 minutes

1 pound no-salt-added farmer cheese

2 eggs

½ cup all-purpose flour, sifted

½ teaspoon salt

sour cream, to serve

1. Boil a large pot of salted water.

2. Mix the farmer cheese and the eggs in a large bowl.

3. Add the flour and salt, and mix thoroughly into a dough. If the dough is too soft, add a little more flour.

4. Roll the dough into a thin tube, then cut into pieces.

5. Drop the dumplings into the boiling water. When the dumplings float to the top they're ready, about 5 to 7 minutes.

6. Remove the dumplings from the water with a skimmer spoon or slotted spoon, and serve with a dollop of sour cream.

Nutrition facts per serving
215 calories | 13.6 g total fat | 7.7 g saturated fat | 1.4 g carbohydrate | 0 g fiber | 19.5 g protein | 0.49 mg iron | 19 mg calcium

Creamy Fruit Salad Snack

Yield: 4 servings   **Prep time:** 15 minutes

1 cup low-fat vanilla yogurt	1 apple, diced
juice of ½ lemon	1 pear, diced
½ teaspoon vanilla extract	1 cup quartered strawberries
½ teaspoon ground cinnamon	1 cup diced pineapple

1. In a small bowl, blend together the yogurt, lemon juice, vanilla, and cinnamon.

2. In a medium bowl, toss together the fruit.

3. Pour the yogurt mixture over the fruit, mix well, and enjoy!

Nutrition facts per serving
130 calories | 0.9 g total fat | 0.3 g saturated fat | 31.2 g carbohydrate | 4.2 g fiber | 2.1 g protein | 0.41 mg iron | 85 mg calcium

Mojito Fruit Salad Parfait Snack

Yield: 6 servings   **Prep time:** 15 minutes

juice of 1 lime

1 tablespoon finely chopped fresh mint

1 apple, diced

1 pear, diced

1 cup seedless purple grapes

1 orange, peeled, with each segment cut in half

¾ cup fresh blueberries

¾ cup fresh blackberries

4 cups nonfat plain Greek yogurt

1 cup puffed rice cereal

1. In a small bowl, whisk together the lime juice and mint. Set aside.

2. In a medium bowl, combine the fruits.

3. Pour the lime-mint mixture over the fruit and mix well.

4. In short glass tumblers, place a layer of yogurt followed by a layer of fruit. Continue to alternate layers.

5. Top each tumbler with the cereal.

Nutrition facts per serving
149 calories | 0.2 g total fat | 0 g saturated fat | 25.5 g carbohydrate | 3.8 g fiber | 12.1 g protein | 0.31 mg iron | 183 mg calcium

Tzatziki Toasts

Yield: 4 servings   **Prep time:** 20 minutes

1 large cucumber, peeled and deseeded, grated

1 cup low-fat plain Greek yogurt

2 cloves garlic, finely minced

1 tablespoon extra virgin olive oil

2 teaspoons lemon juice

1 tablespoon finely minced fresh dill

salt, to taste

black pepper, to taste

4 slices whole grain bread

3 radishes, thinly sliced, to top

1 large tomato, thinly sliced, to top

15 kalamata olives, pitted and halved, to top

1. Place the cucumber into a fine-mesh sieve over a bowl to allow the water to drain. Add a pinch of salt to the cucumber to help speed up this process.

2. In a medium bowl, combine the yogurt, garlic, olive oil, lemon juice, dill, salt, and pepper.

3. Add the cucumber and mix well.

4. Toast the bread in a toaster.

5. Smear a layer of the mixture over each slice of bread and top with the radishes, tomato, and kalamata olives.

Nutrition facts per serving
246 calories | 10 g total fat | 0.6 g saturated fat | 28.9 g carbohydrate | 1.9 g fiber | 11.6 g protein | 0.74 mg iron | 94 mg calcium

Polenta Caprese Salad

Yield: 5 servings   **Prep time:** 15 minutes   **Cook time:** 20 minutes

4 teaspoons olive oil, divided

1 (18-ounce) package Trader Joe's organic precooked polenta, sliced into 18 slices

salt, to taste

2 large tomatoes, sliced

6 ounces fresh mozzarella, thinly sliced

1 small bunch fresh basil, stems discarded

1 tablespoon extra virgin olive oil

3 tablespoons balsamic glaze

black pepper, to taste

1. Preheat the oven to 400°F.

2. Line a baking sheet with parchment paper and spread with 2 teaspoons olive oil.

3. Place the polenta slices on the baking sheet.

4. Brush the remaining 2 teaspoons of olive oil on the top of each polenta slice and season with salt.

5. Place into the oven and bake for 20 minutes until golden. Set aside to cool.

6. When cool, arrange a platter with alternating layers of polenta, tomato, mozzarella, and basil leaves.

7. Drizzle with the extra virgin olive oil and balsamic glaze, then sprinkle with a little salt and pepper.

Nutrition facts per serving
237 calories | 12.3 g total fat | 4.5 g saturated fat | 25.1 g carbohydrate | 4 g fiber | 7.9 g protein | 0.86 mg iron | 202 mg calcium

Kani Salad

You may have seen kani salad on the menu at a Japanese restaurant, so it may come as no surprise that "kani" is a Japanese word meaning crab. More often than not, imitation crab meat is used in place of the real thing. It is very easy to handle and is a more budget-friendly option.

Yield: 4 servings   **Prep time:** 15 minutes

1 pound imitation crab meat, flaked

2 ribs celery, thinly sliced

2 cucumbers, peeled and deseeded, thinly sliced

¼ cup chopped fresh parsley

2 tablespoons mayonnaise

1 tablespoon sriracha

1 tablespoon mustard

chopped scallions, for garnish

1. In a medium bowl, combine the imitation crab meat, celery, cucumbers, and parsley.

2. In a small bowl, mix together the mayonnaise, sriracha, and mustard.

3. Add the mayonnaise mixture to the crab meat and mix well.

4. Sprinkle with scallions before serving.

Nutrition facts per serving
194 calories| 6.4 g total fat | 0.8 g saturated fat | 25 g carbohydrate | 0.6 g fiber | 9.9 g protein | 0.18 mg iron | 19 mg calcium

Roasted Endive

Yield: 2 servings   **Prep time:** 10 minutes   **Cook time:** 45 minutes to 1 hour

3 endives, halved lengthwise

1½ tablespoons olive oil

salt, to taste

black pepper, to taste

1. Preheat the oven to 350°F.

2. On a parchment-lined baking sheet, place the endives and drizzle with the olive oil.

3. Season with salt and pepper.

4. Bake for approximately 30 minutes, flip, and roast for another 15 to 30 minutes until the endive is golden and tender.

5. Serve hot.

Nutrition facts per serving
96 calories | 10.1 g total fat | 1.4 g saturated fat | 0 g carbohydrate | 0 g fiber | 0 g protein | 0.07 mg iron | 0 mg calcium

Cheesy Broccoli

This side dish is a good source of protein. While not being high in iron, it offers a solid dose of calcium alongside some curcumin to help inhibit iron absorption.

Yield: 2 servings   **Prep time:** 10 minutes   **Cook time:** 15 minutes

2 cups broccoli florets

½ cup nonfat plain Greek yogurt

¼ teaspoon ground turmeric

¼ teaspoon ground cumin

¼ teaspoon ground coriander

¼ teaspoon smoked paprika

¼ teaspoon salt

¼ teaspoon black pepper

3 ounces reduced-fat cheddar cheese, shredded

1. Preheat the oven to 400°F.

2. On the stovetop, steam the broccoli in a steamer until it is tender but still firm, about 5 minutes.

3. In a small bowl, combine the yogurt, turmeric, cumin, coriander, smoked paprika, salt, and pepper.

4. Transfer the broccoli to a 3-quart baking dish, pour in the yogurt mixture, mix together, and top with the cheese.

5. Place the dish into the oven. Bake for approximately 10 minutes until the cheese is melted.

6. Serve hot.

Nutrition facts per serving
168 calories | 9.2 g total fat | 3.8 g saturated fat | 6.2 g carbohydrate | 0.9 g fiber | 16.6 g protein | 0.40 mg iron | 427 mg calcium

Mixed Fruit Kompot

Kompot is a popular, fruity Russian beverage. As a Russian-American, I favored this drink growing up; it's essentially a refreshing homemade juice and snack all rolled into one! This simple recipe is best enjoyed alone because it increases the absorption of iron when taken with food.

Yield: 8 servings   **Prep time:** 15 minutes   **Cook time:** 30 minutes

3 pears, cored and quartered

4 apples, cored and quartered

5 plums, pitted and quartered

2 tablespoons sugar

juice of ½ lemon

1. Place the fruits into a large pot and fill with enough water to cover the fruits.

2. Bring the water to a boil, cover with the lid, and allow the fruit to simmer on low to medium heat until tender, roughly 30 minutes.

3. When the fruit is tender, stir in the sugar and mix until dissolved.

4. After stirring in the sugar, strain the kompot through a sieve and set the liquid aside to cool.

5. Chop the cooked fruit into bite-size pieces and then return it with the drained liquid to the pot.

6. Once the fruit and liquid are cooled, stir in the lemon juice and refrigerate.

7. Serve chilled.

Nutrition facts per serving
109 calories | 0.1 g total fat | 0 g saturated fat | 29.3 g carbohydrate | 5.4 g fiber | 0.2 g protein | 0.36 mg iron | 44 mg calcium

Zucchini Salad

Yield: 2 servings   **Prep time:** 25 minutes

¾ cup low-fat cottage cheese

1 tablespoon chopped
fresh chives

1 large carrot, shredded

black pepper, to taste

2 large zucchinis,
sliced into ribbons

2 tablespoons chopped
fresh parsley

1. Add the cottage cheese, chives, carrot, and black pepper to a blender and mix until smooth.

2. Pour the cottage cheese mixture over the zucchini ribbons, toss, and top with parsley.

Nutrition facts per serving
118 calories | 2.1 g total fat | 1.1 g saturated fat | 12.8 g carbohydrate | 3.2 g fiber | 13.6 g protein | 0.99 mg iron | 130 mg calcium

Tofu Salad

I've listed this as a salad, but you can also use it to make sand-wiches with whole wheat bread.

Yield: 4 servings   **Prep time:** 15 minutes

12 ounces firm silken tofu, drained

¼ cup low-fat plain yogurt

2 tablespoons finely chopped chives

1 tablespoon finely chopped fresh dill

1 rib celery, finely chopped

1 tablespoon Dijon mustard

½ teaspoon ground turmeric

salt, to taste

black pepper, to taste

1. In a large bowl, mash the tofu with a fork.

2. Add the yogurt, chives, dill, celery, mustard, and turmeric. Season with salt and pepper, and mix gently.

3. Enjoy!

Nutrition facts per serving
73 calories | 5.2 g total fat | 0.3 g saturated fat | 4.6 g carbohydrate | 0.2 g fiber | 5.8 g protein | 1 mg iron | 69 mg calcium

Salmon Salad

Do not discard the soft, calcium-rich bones! Once mashed with a fork, they are unnoticeable and play a part in inhibiting the absorption of iron.

Yield: 2 servings **Prep time:** 15 minutes

1 (7.5-ounce) can wild Alaskan salmon with the bones

2 cups baby arugula leaves

1½ tablespoons capers

1 tablespoon avocado oil mayonnaise

black pepper, to taste

1. Drain the liquid from the canned salmon. Remove the skin. Mash the salmon with a fork (the bones are very soft).

2. Mix in the remaining ingredients.

3. Enjoy with whole wheat bread or whole wheat crackers.

Nutrition facts per serving
210 calories | 14.5 g total fat | 2.5 g saturated fat | 1.3 g carbohydrate | 0.5 g fiber | 21.1 g protein | 1.08 mg iron | 221 mg calcium

Mixed Leaf Caesar

Yield: 4 servings   **Prep time:** 15 minutes   **Cook time:** 10 minutes

2 slices whole wheat
bread, cubed

2 tablespoons olive oil

1 teaspoon garlic powder

½ teaspoon ground turmeric

salt, to taste

black pepper, to taste

1 cup spinach leaves

1 cup chopped romaine lettuce

Caesar Dressing (page 82)

1. Preheat the oven to 400°F.

2. On a parchment paper–lined baking sheet, mix together the bread cubes, olive oil, garlic powder, turmeric, salt, and pepper.

3. Spread into one layer, so the bread cubes do not overlap.

4. Bake until toasted, approximately 10 minutes.

5. Place the spinach and lettuce into a bowl. Top with the croutons, drizzle with the Caesar dressing, and toss. Sprinkle with black pepper before serving.

Nutrition facts per serving
101 calories | 7.4 g total fat | 1 g saturated fat | 7.9 g carbohydrate |
1.5 g fiber | 1.7 g protein | 0.92 mg iron | 19 mg calcium

Caesar Dressing

Yield: 4 servings   **Prep time:** 5 minutes

1 small clove garlic

1 teaspoon capers

1 tablespoon
Parmesan cheese

1 tablespoon low-fat
plain Greek yogurt

1 tablespoon olive oil

1 teaspoon Dijon mustard

Place the garlic, capers, Parmesan cheese, Greek yogurt, olive oil, and mustard in a blender, and blend until smooth. If the dressing is too thick, add a small amount of warm water.

Nutrition facts per serving
57 calories | 4.9 g total fat | 0.9 g saturated fat | 4.4 g carbohydrate | 2.3 g fiber | 2.6 g protein | 1.28 mg iron | 55 mg calcium

Lunch

Smoky Lentil Burgers

The black tea is a star ingredient here. Not only does it give this recipe an iron-inhibiting dose of polyphenols, but it also adds a delicious smoky element to these burgers. The inclusion of phosvitin and phytate-rich ingredients doesn't hurt either!

Yield: 8 (1-burger) servings   **Prep time:** 20 minutes
Cook time: 1 hour, 15 minutes

2 tea bags black tea	¼ teaspoon salt
8 ounces boiling water	½ teaspoon garlic powder
½ cup rinsed red lentils	½ teaspoon onion powder
1 medium carrot, diced	1 teaspoon smoked paprika
½ medium yellow onion, diced	½ cup bread crumbs
2 eggs	

1. Add the tea bags to the boiling water and allow them to steep for 6 minutes.

2. Discard the tea bags. In a medium saucepan over medium-high heat, combine the lentils with the tea, bring to a boil, lower the heat to medium-low, cover, and simmer for 25 to 30 minutes until the lentils are soft.

3. Once the lentils are done cooking, let sit covered for 10 minutes.

4. In a medium pan, sauté the carrot and onion over medium heat.

5. Place the lentils, sautéed vegetables, and eggs into a blender or food processor. Blend until almost smooth.

6. Pour into a bowl and add the salt, garlic powder, onion powder, and smoked paprika. Mix well.

7. Mix in the bread crumbs and let stand for 3 to 5 minutes to thicken.

8. Form the mixture into ⅓-inch-thick patties, place in a 12-inch skillet on medium-low heat, and cook for approximately 3 minutes on each side.

9. Serve alongside a salad or enjoy as a sandwich.

Nutrition facts per serving
96 calories | 1.6 g total fat | 0.4 g saturated fat | 14.6 g carbohydrate | 1.9 g fiber | 5.8 g protein | 1.44 mg iron | 27 mg calcium

Macaroni Casserole

Sometimes you just crave comfort food. This casserole is a fraction of the calories and fat of the typical version while still offering a decent amount of protein, some nonheme iron, and inhibitors like curcumin, calcium, and phosvitin.

Yield: 12 servings   **Prep time:** 10 minutes   **Cook time:** 50 minutes

1 pound elbow macaroni	¼ teaspoon ground cumin
1 cup evaporated nonfat milk	¼ teaspoon chili powder
½ cup unsweetened vanilla almond milk	1 egg
8 ounces soft goat cheese	pinch of salt
¼ teaspoon ground turmeric	½ cup shredded cheddar cheese

1. Prepare the macaroni according to package instructions. Drain and set aside in a large bowl.

2. Preheat the oven to 350°F.

3. In a small saucepan, heat the evaporated milk, almond milk, and goat cheese until the cheese dissolves. Stir in the turmeric, cumin, and chili powder.

4. Pour the milk-cheese mixture over the cooked macaroni and stir to combine.

5. In a small bowl, whisk the egg with a pinch of salt.

6. Stir the egg into the macaroni.

7. Spread the macaroni mixture into a 3-quart glass baking dish and sprinkle the top with the shredded cheese.

8. Bake for 30 minutes, until the cheese melts and the top is golden.

9. Serve immediately.

Nutrition facts per serving
224 calories | 6.7 g total fat | 3.9 g saturated fat | 31 g carbohydrate | 1.4 g fiber | 11.2 g protein | 1.71 mg iron | 128 mg calcium

Mushroom Soup

Yield: 8 servings   **Prep time:** 30 minutes
Cook time: 1 hour, 10 minutes

2 ounces dried porcini
mushrooms

3 cups boiling water

1 medium yellow onion, diced

2 tablespoons olive oil

¼ celery root, diced

3 ribs celery, diced

1 large carrot, shredded

1½ teaspoons salt, divided

1 teaspoon black pepper

10 ounces fresh button
mushrooms, sliced

4 tea bags black tea

1 cup dried barley

dill, finely chopped, for garnish

nonfat plain Greek
yogurt, to serve

1. Soak the porcini mushrooms in the boiling water for 20 minutes.
Drain the porcinis and reserve the liquid for later use.

2. In a large pot, sauté the onion in the olive oil, stirring
occasionally, until the onion is translucent, about 5 minutes.

3. Add the celery root, celery, carrot, 1 teaspoon salt, and pepper,
stirring until softened, about 10 minutes.

4. Add the button mushrooms to the vegetable mixture, season
with the remaining ½ teaspoon salt, and when tender, add the
softened porcini mushrooms into the pot with the liquid they were
steeping in.

5. Add water, filling the pot three-quarters full.

6. Simmer, with the pot partially covered, for 30 minutes.

7. While the soup simmers, place the tea bags into the pot,
removing them after 5 minutes.

8. Add the barley and cook about 15 minutes with the cover ajar until the grain is tender.

9. Garnish with a sprinkling of dill and serve with a dollop of Greek yogurt.

Nutrition facts per serving
186 calories | 4.6 g total fat | 0.6 g saturated fat | 29.4 g carbohydrate | 5.2 g fiber | 8.6 g protein | 0.9 mg iron, 46 mg calcium

Vegan Nourish Bowl

Yield: 1 serving   **Prep time:** 10 minutes

½ cup cooked long grain brown rice

½ cup canned chickpeas, drained and rinsed

1 tablespoon chopped fresh scallions

¼ cup sliced green bell pepper

1 cucumber, diced

1 teaspoon chopped fresh cilantro

Green Goddess Dressing (page 91)

Place all ingredients into a bowl, mix together, and drizzle with Green Goddess Dressing.

Nutrition facts per serving
275 calories | 3 g total fat | 0.2 g saturated fat | 57.5 g carbohydrate | 10.6 g fiber | 11.5 g protein | 3.44 g iron | 133 mg calcium

Green Goddess Dressing

This fresh-tasting dressing pairs nicely with the Vegan Nourish Bowl but can also be used to top other dishes like fresh salads.

Yield: 6 servings   **Prep time:** 10 minutes

2 whole scallions

⅓ cup low-fat plain Greek yogurt

1 clove garlic

¼ cup extra virgin olive oil

½ cup coarsely chopped cilantro

1 teaspoon salt

¼ teaspoon black pepper

1 tablespoon lemon juice

¼ cup water

Place all ingredients into a blender. Blend until creamy. For a thinner consistency, add more water.

Nutrition facts per serving
93 calories | 9.6 g total fat | 1.5 g saturated fat | 1.1 g carbohydrate | 0.1 g fiber | 1.5 g protein | 0.2 mg iron | 21 mg calcium

Spring Rolls

When eating poultry, go for white meat chicken and turkey as it contains less iron than dark meat. As a rule of thumb, the darker the hue of the meat the higher it will be in iron while the lightest cuts will be the lowest.

Yield: 4 (2-roll) servings **Prep time:** 25 minutes
Cook time: 40 minutes

2 (6-ounce) skinless, boneless chicken breasts

1 cup black tea

2 tablespoons olive oil, divided

salt, to taste

black pepper, to taste

1 carrot, julienned

1 green bell pepper, julienned

2 whole scallions, julienned

2 cloves garlic, minced

⅛ teaspoon ground ginger

½ cup shredded cabbage

1 tablespoon chopped fresh basil

1 tablespoon reduced-sodium soy sauce

1 teaspoon sesame oil

8 rice paper wrappers

Peanut Sauce (page 94)

1. Marinate the chicken breasts in tea overnight.

2. Preheat the oven to 400°F.

3. Pour out all of the liquid. Pat the chicken dry.

4. Place the chicken breasts on a baking sheet lined with parchment paper.

5. Rub the chicken with 1 tablespoon olive oil and season with salt and pepper to taste.

6. Bake for approximately 30 to 40 minutes, until the chicken is cooked through. Set aside to cool.

7. While the chicken is baking, add the remaining tablespoon of olive oil to a 12-inch pan over medium-high heat.

8. Add the carrot, bell pepper, scallions, garlic, ginger, and cabbage, and sauté until slightly tender, about 10 minutes.

9. Stir in the basil, soy sauce, sesame oil, and pepper. Remove from the heat.

10. Once the chicken has cooled, slice it into strips.

11. Fill a shallow pan with warm water. Place the rice paper into the warm water for 5 seconds, then place on a cutting board.

12. Spoon one-eighth of the filling into the wrapper, drizzle with Peanut Sauce, add one-eighth of the chicken, and roll it up.

Tip: For a simple way to secure the roll, place the filling toward the bottom of the rice paper wrapper. Fold over on each side and then roll upward.

Nutrition facts per serving
234 calories | 11 g total fat | 1.1 g saturated fat | 13.2 g carbohydrate | 1.5 g fiber | 22.2 g protein | 1.73 mg iron | 33 mg calcium

Peanut Sauce

Yield: 4 servings   **Prep time:** 5 minutes

1½ teaspoons sriracha

1 tablespoon reduced-
sodium soy sauce

1 teaspoon sesame oil

2 tablespoons peanut butter

2 teaspoons honey

Whisk all of the ingredients together in a bowl.

Nutrition facts per serving
66 calories | 5.3 g total fat | 1 g saturated fat | 3.4 g carbohydrate |
0.5 g fiber | 2.3 g protein | 0.18 mg iron | 0 mg calcium

Eggplant Rollups

Yield: 4 servings   **Prep time:** 25 minutes   **Cook time:** 30 minutes

2 tablespoons olive oil, divided

1 eggplant, sliced lengthwise into ⅛- to ¼-inch-thick slices

salt, to taste

black pepper, to taste

1 small yellow onion, diced

1 medium carrot, shredded

1 red, orange, or yellow bell pepper, diced

½ teaspoon MSG-free Vegeta seasoning

¼ cup low-fat plain Greek yogurt

2 cloves garlic, crushed or finely minced

1. Preheat the oven to 400°F. Line a baking sheet with parchment paper and drizzle with 1 tablespoon olive oil.

2. Season the eggplant with salt and pepper, place on the baking sheet, and bake until soft, about 10 to 20 minutes (time will vary depending on the thickness of the slices). When done, set aside to cool.

3. In a 12-inch pan over medium-high heat, add the remaining olive oil, onion, carrot, and bell pepper. Season with the Vegeta and some pepper, then sauté until the vegetables are tender, about 10 minutes. Set aside to cool.

4. Mix the Greek yogurt and garlic together in a small bowl.

5. Spread a teaspoon of the garlicky Greek yogurt over each eggplant slice.

6. Add a teaspoon of the sautéed vegetables and beginning at the narrow end, roll up the eggplant and place on a serving platter.

Nutrition facts per serving
131 calories | 7.6 g total fat | 1.3 g saturated fat | 12.7 g carbohydrate | 5.1 g fiber | 5 g protein | 1.15 mg iron | 80 mg calcium

Green Bean Frittata

Yield: 4 servings   **Prep time:** 15 minutes   **Cook time:** 20 minutes

2 teaspoons olive oil

⅓ cup diced onion

6 eggs

1 ounce Parmesan
cheese, grated

salt, to taste

black pepper, to taste

½ cup chopped roasted
green beans

1. Preheat the oven to 500°F or to high under the broil setting.

2. Add the olive oil to a 12-inch pan over medium-high heat.

3. Add the onion and sauté until soft and translucent, about
6 minutes.

4. While the onion is sautéing, whisk together the eggs, Parmesan
cheese, salt, and pepper in a medium bowl.

5. When the onion is soft, add the green beans to the onion and
sauté for another 3 minutes.

6. Pour the egg mixture into the pan and stir. Cook for about
5 minutes or until it's about three-quarters set.

7. Broil in the oven for 3 minutes.

8. Remove from the pan, cut, and serve immediately.

Nutrition facts per serving
171 calories | 11.4 g total fat | 3.9 g saturated fat | 2.6 g carbohydrate |
0.2 g fiber | 12.3 g protein | 1.42 mg iron | 124 mg calcium

Dinner

Caramelized Onion Pizza

Use a ready-made pizza crust or make your own.

Yield: 6 servings   **Prep time:** 10 minutes   **Cook time:** 40 minutes

3 tablespoons olive oil, divided

2 medium white onions, thinly sliced

salt, to taste

black pepper, to taste

1 whole wheat ready-made pizza crust

5 ounces goat cheese

1. Preheat the oven to 400°F.

2. Add 2 tablespoons olive oil and the onion to a 10-inch pan over medium-high heat. Season with salt and pepper, and sauté until the onion is soft and golden, about 10 minutes.

3. Reduce the heat to low and continue to cook until the onion is darker brown, about 20 minutes.

4. Coat the pizza crust with the remaining tablespoon of olive oil. Spread an even layer of onion over the crust, then top with crumbled goat cheese. Season with a little more pepper.

5. Bake on the middle rack until the crust is golden, approximately 10 minutes. (Time may vary if homemade pizza dough is used.)

Nutrition facts per serving
208 calories | 12.7 g total fat | 4.3 g saturated fat | 14.2 g carbohydrate | 2.5 g fiber | 7.2 g protein | 1.28 mg iron | 46 mg calcium

Pesto Pasta

This recipe is a great example of how to incorporate a high-iron vegetable like spinach into your diet. Enjoy it raw and feel free to incorporate other ingredients that contain inhibitors such as calcium and phytates.

Yield: 6 servings   **Prep time:** 15 minutes   **Cook time:** 10 minutes

12 ounces whole wheat spaghetti

2 tablespoons almonds

2 large cloves garlic

½ cup grated Parmigiano-Reggiano cheese

1 cup raw spinach leaves

1 cup fresh basil leaves

¼ cup extra virgin olive oil

salt, to taste

black pepper, to taste

Parmesan cheese, to serve (optional)

1. Prepare the spaghetti according to package directions. Once cooked, reserve ½ cup of the cooking liquid and discard the rest.

2. To make pesto, in a food processor, pulse the almonds and garlic until finely ground. Add the Parmigiano-Reggiano cheese, spinach, and basil, and blend. While blending, add the olive oil in a slow stream. Blend until the mixture is nearly smooth, then season with salt and pepper.

3. Toss the spaghetti with the cooking liquid and the pesto.

4. Top with a little Parmesan cheese, if desired.

Nutrition facts per serving
325 calories | 13.3 g total fat | 2.9 g saturated fat | 44.3 g carbohydrate | 0.9 g fiber | 11.8 g protein | 2.32 mg iron | 102 mg calcium

Creamy Cod

Yield: 8 servings   **Prep time:** 15 minutes   **Cook time:** 30 minutes

4 (4-ounce) cod fillets

salt, to taste

2 tablespoons olive oil

For the cream sauce:

2 tablespoons softened butter

2 tablespoons cornstarch

1 cup 2% reduced-fat milk

¼ cup grated
Parmesan cheese

3 cloves garlic, crushed

½ cup whole wheat
seasoned bread crumbs

1 teaspoon ground turmeric

salt, to taste

black pepper, to taste

1. Preheat the oven to 400°F.

2. Spread a light layer of olive oil on the bottom of a 3-quart baking dish. Place the cod in the dish and season each fillet with salt.

3. Mix together the 2 tablespoons olive oil and the garlic, and distribute evenly over each fillet. Top with seasoned bread crumbs.

4. To make the cream sauce, melt the butter in a medium saucepan. Stir in the cornstarch, whisking to incorporate. Whisking continually, add the milk until well mixed. Stir in the Parmesan cheese. Let sit over low heat until the consistency of a cream sauce, about 2 minutes. Season with turmeric, salt, and pepper, and mix well.

5. Pour the sauce over the fish and bake for approximately 20 to 25 minutes until the fish is opaque and flaky.

Nutrition facts per serving
183 calories | 10 g total fat | 3.5 g saturated fat | 7.9 g carbohydrate | 0.7 g fiber | 15 g protein | 0.54 mg iron | 96 mg calcium

Earthy Haddock

Although the iron in fish is better absorbed than the iron from a plant source, fish contains far less iron than red meat. It is also an excellent source of protein and heart healthy fats known as omega-3 fatty acids. Try to include three servings of fish in your diet weekly!

Yield: 4 servings   **Prep time:** 10 minutes   **Cook time:** 25 minutes

4 (4-ounce) haddock fillets	½ teaspoon ground ginger
1 teaspoon smoked paprika	salt, to taste
1 teaspoon ground coriander	black pepper, to taste
1 teaspoon ground turmeric	2 tablespoons olive oil

1. Preheat the oven to 400°F.

2. Spread a light layer of olive oil on the bottom of a 3-quart baking dish. Place the haddock in the dish.

3. Combine the paprika, coriander, turmeric, ginger, salt, and pepper in a small bowl.

4. Rub the olive oil on the haddock, then evenly distribute the seasoning mixture over each fillet.

5. Bake for 18 minutes and then broil for another 2 to 3 minutes. The fish should be flaky once cooked through.

Nutrition facts per serving
161 calories | 7.7 g total fat | 0.9 g saturated fat | 1.1 g carbohydrate | 0.4 g fiber | 0.47 mg iron | 4 mg calcium

Quinoa (Bean-less) Chili

This dish is a great option for your Meatless Monday as quinoa is a whole grain that also happens to be a complete protein. There are also phytates and polyphenols in this dish to help keep the iron in check.

Yield: 3 servings   **Prep time:** 15 minutes   **Cook time:** 30 minutes

1 tablespoon olive oil

1 large yellow onion, chopped

1 large carrot, chopped

2 ribs celery, chopped

3 cloves garlic, minced

salt, to taste

black pepper, to taste

1 (32-ounce) carton vegetable broth

1 (14.5-ounce) can fire-roasted diced tomatoes

½ cup quinoa

1 teaspoon chili powder

1 teaspoon unsweetened cocoa powder

1 tablespoon finely ground coffee

1 teaspoon cumin

nonfat plain Greek yogurt, to serve (optional)

chopped cilantro, to serve (optional)

1. Warm the olive oil in a large saucepan over medium-high heat.

2. Add the onion, carrot, celery, and garlic, then season with salt and pepper. Sauté until the onion softens, about 10 minutes.

3. Lower to medium heat and add the vegetable broth, diced tomatoes, and quinoa. Stir to combine, then mix in the chili powder, cocoa powder, ground coffee, and cumin.

4. Cover and simmer until the quinoa is cooked, about 20 minutes.

5. Serve with a dollop of Greek yogurt and cilantro, if using.

Nutrition facts per serving
248 calories | 6.9 g total fat | 0.8 g saturated fat | 40.4 g carbohydrates |
12.7 g fiber | 6 g protein | 3.73 mg iron | 76 mg calcium

Stroganoff Chicken Meatballs

This recipe includes dairy and whole grains to help inhibit the absorption of iron. Enjoy with a cup of tea to help reduce the absorption of iron further.

Yield: 6 (5-meatball) servings **Prep time:** 30 minutes
Cook time: 1 hour

1 pound ground chicken

¾ cup whole wheat
bread crumbs

¾ cup low-fat milk

1 egg

2 medium onions, finely
chopped, divided

salt, to taste

black pepper, to taste

2 tablespoons olive oil

8 ounces white
mushrooms, sliced

2 cloves garlic

3 tablespoons all-
purpose flour

1 (32-ounce) carton
chicken broth

2 tablespoons sour cream

¼ cup 2% evaporated milk

2 tablespoons chopped
fresh parsley

1. Preheat the oven to 400°F. Line a baking sheet with parchment paper and coat with a little cooking spray.

2. In a large bowl, combine the chicken, bread crumbs, milk, egg, 1 chopped onion, salt, and pepper.

3. Roll the mixture into 30 small meatballs. Place on the baking sheet.

4. Bake for 20 to 25 minutes. They do not need to be completely cooked as they will continue to cook in the stroganoff sauce.

5. In a large skillet or pot, heat the olive oil on medium-high heat.

6. Sauté the remaining onion until tender, about 5 minutes.

7. Add the mushrooms and garlic, salt, and pepper, and cook until the mixture is golden brown, about 10 minutes.

8. Add the flour and mix well until you can no longer see the flour. Pour in the chicken broth and mix very well. Allow the sauce to simmer on low to medium heat, about 5 minutes.

9. Once the sauce thickens, add the sour cream and evaporated milk. Mix with a whisk until smooth.

10. Place the meatballs into the sauce and cook until well done, about 8 minutes.

11. Mix in the parsley, and serve hot.

Nutrition facts per serving
270 calories | 12.7 g total fat | 3.8 g saturated fat | 18.9 g carbohydrate | 2.3 g fiber | 20.5 g protein | 2.12 mg iron | 119 mg calcium

Roasted Vegetable Medley

This side dish will give a nice boost of calcium to any meal!

Yield: 3 servings   **Prep time:** 20 minutes   **Cook time:** 45 minutes

2 large carrots, halved and cut into 1-inch pieces

1 cup halved Brussels sprouts

1 medium red onion, halved and cut into 1-inch pieces

medium yellow onion, halved and cut into 1-inch pieces

1 cup cauliflower florets

2 tablespoons olive oil

½ teaspoon dried rosemary

½ teaspoon dried oregano

¾ teaspoon dried basil

salt, to taste

black pepper, to taste

1. Preheat the oven to 400°F.

2. In a large bowl, combine the carrots, Brussels sprouts, onions, and cauliflower, and toss them with the olive oil, rosemary, oregano, basil, salt, and pepper. If the vegetables feel dry, add another tablespoon of oil.

3. Spread the vegetables on a parchment paper–lined baking sheet and place on the center rack in the oven.

4. Bake for 45 minutes, stirring the vegetables every 15 minutes.

5. Season with a pinch of salt once roasted.

Nutrition facts per serving
153 calories | 9.2 g total fat | 1.3 g saturated fat | 15.4 g carbohydrate | 3.2 g fiber | 2.6 g protein | 0.76 mg iron | 336 mg calcium

Shiitake BLT

This is a vegetarian spin on the classic bacon, lettuce, and tomato sandwich. Think more along the lines of butterhead lettuce tomato in this case. This version, while sans bacon, is just as savory and crispy because of the way in which the mushrooms are prepared. Get ready to be pleasantly surprised!

Yield: 2 servings   **Prep time:** 10 minutes   **Cook time:** 12 minutes

6 large shiitake mushrooms, stems removed, caps sliced

1 tablespoon olive oil

salt, to taste

black pepper, to taste

1 whole wheat pita

2 teaspoons mustard

4 leaves butterhead lettuce

½ heirloom tomato, sliced ¼-inch thick

2 ounces smoked Gouda, sliced

1. Preheat the oven to 375°F.

2. On a parchment paper–lined baking sheet, toss the mushrooms with the olive oil, salt, and pepper.

3. Bake until crispy, about 12 minutes. Check on the mushrooms throughout to ensure they do not burn.

4. Cut the pita in half and open the pocket.

5. Spread 1 teaspoon of mustard in the pocket of each pita half.

6. Fill each pita half with lettuce, tomato, shiitake mushrooms, and smoked Gouda.

Nutrition facts per serving
268 calories | 14.5 g total fat | 5.9 g saturated fat | 26.4 g carbohydrate | 3.2 g fiber | 10.9 g protein | 1 mg iron | 342 mg calcium

Bean Chili

This may appear to be very high in iron, but legumes contain phytates, which inhibit the absorption of iron. Other inhibitors present in this recipe are polyphenols and curcumin.

Yield: 2 servings   **Prep time:** 20 minutes
Cook time: 1 hour, 45 minutes

5 tea bags black tea

3 cups boiling water

½ cup dry pinto beans, rinsed, soaked overnight, and drained

1 tablespoon olive oil

1 medium onion, chopped

3 cloves garlic, minced

1 large carrot, finely chopped

1 rib celery, finely chopped

1 teaspoon ground cumin

1 teaspoon smoked paprika

black pepper, to taste

salt, to taste

½ teaspoon cayenne pepper

½ teaspoon ground turmeric

16 ounces vegetable broth

¼ cup chopped fresh cilantro, for garnish

1. In a medium saucepan, place the tea bags in the boiling water for 6 minutes.

2. Remove the tea bags and add the beans to the saucepan. Cook the beans in the tea for about 1 hour over medium heat.

3. In a separate large pot, heat the olive oil over medium-high heat.

4. Sauté the onion until translucent, about 5 minutes. Add the garlic, carrot, and celery, and sauté until tender, about 10 minutes.

5. Season with cumin, smoked paprika, black pepper, salt, cayenne pepper, and turmeric, and stir to combine.

6. Add the beans. Pour in the vegetable broth and simmer on low to medium heat, stirring occasionally for at least 30 minutes.

7. Serve in bowls and garnish with cilantro.

Nutrition facts per serving
185 calories | 7.2 g total fat | 0.9 g saturated fat | 35.6 g carbohydrate |
16.9 g fiber | 9.2 g protein | 4.75 mg iron | 94 mg calcium

Perfectly Marinated Chicken

Yield: 8 servings   **Prep time:** 15 minutes plus overnight to marinate
Cook time: varies

1 cup low-fat plain
Greek yogurt

1 tablespoon olive oil

2 cloves garlic, minced

1 teaspoon chili powder

1 teaspoon smoked paprika

salt, to taste

black pepper, to taste

2 pounds skinless,
boneless chicken breast

1. Mix the yogurt, oil, garlic, chili powder, smoked paprika, salt, and pepper in a small bowl.

2. Place the chicken in a sealable container and pour in the marinade, ensuring that the chicken is coated well.

3. Seal the container and refrigerate overnight.

4. Bake at 375°F for approximately 30 to 40 minutes or grill for roughly 10 minutes per side, or until cooked through.

5. Let the chicken rest for 5 minutes before serving.

Nutrition facts per serving
177 calories | 6.1 g total fat | 0.5 g saturated fat | 1.3 g carbohydrate | 0.1 g fiber | 30.9 g protein | 1.26 mg iron | 45 mg calcium

Coffee-Rubbed Salmon

Yield: 4 servings   **Prep time:** 10 minutes   **Cook time:** 20 minutes

2 teaspoons avocado oil

1 pound skin-on salmon, cut into 4 fillets

1 tablespoon finely ground coffee

2 teaspoons ground coriander

½ teaspoon ground turmeric

½ teaspoon chili powder

2 teaspoons smoked paprika

1 teaspoon garlic powder

salt, to taste

1. Preheat the oven to 400°F.

2. Line a baking sheet with parchment paper and spread the oil into a thin layer. Place the salmon skin-side down onto the parchment paper.

3. In a small bowl, mix together the coffee, coriander, turmeric, chili powder, smoked paprika, garlic powder, and salt.

4. Sprinkle the salmon evenly with the spice mixture. Using your fingers, rub the mixture into the salmon.

5. Bake the salmon for approximately 18 minutes until the thickest portion of the fish can be easily flaked with a fork. Then broil for 1 to 2 minutes.

6. Serve with your favorite sides, such as string beans and Polenta Caprese Salad (page 73).

Nutrition facts per serving
275 calories | 18.1 g total fat | 3.7 g saturated fat | 3.5 g carbohydrate | 1.6 g fiber | 23.4 g protein | 0.85 mg iron | 11 mg calcium

Beverages

Turmeric Latte

This latte packs a powerful antioxidant punch as spices help reduce inflammation and have been seen to have antibacterial and antiviral qualities. It also offers a good dose of calcium and curcumin to help inhibit the absorption of iron.

Yield: 2 servings   **Prep time:** 5 minutes

¾ cup evaporated fat-free milk

¾ cup water

1 teaspoon ground turmeric

¼ teaspoon ground ginger

pinch of black pepper

pinch of salt

2 teaspoons sugar (optional)

¾ teaspoon ground cinnamon, plus more to serve

1 teaspoon vanilla extract

1. In a medium pot over medium heat, add the milk, water, turmeric, ginger, pepper, salt, sugar (if using), cinnamon, and vanilla. Stir occasionally until the mixture is hot.

2. Remove from the heat and pour the mixture into a blender. Blend on high until well mixed and frothy.

3. Pour into mugs and top with a sprinkle of cinnamon.

Nutrition facts per serving
103 calories | 0.1 g total fat | 0.1 g saturated fat | 17.8 g carbohydrate | 0.7 g fiber | 6.1 g protein | 0.47 mg iron | 249 mg calcium

Iced Chai

Yield: 4 servings   **Prep time:** 10 minutes

4 tea bags chai tea

3 cups boiling water

2 cups unsweetened
vanilla almond milk

ice cubes

4 cinnamon sticks

1. Add the tea bags to the boiling water and let steep for
10 minutes.

2. Remove the tea bags and stir in the almond milk.

3. Chill the chai in the refrigerator.

4. Serve over ice and place a cinnamon stick into each glass
before serving.

Nutrition facts per serving
32 calories | 1.3 g total fat | 0 g saturated fat | 0.5 g carbohydrate |
0.5 g fiber | 0.5 g protein | 0.36 mg iron | 225 mg calcium

Dessert

Chai Tea Ice Cream

This ice cream has all of the notes of a brisk fall day from the warm cinnamon, spicy ginger and peppercorn, and fragrant vanilla, making it an ice cream you can look forward to no matter the season. It also includes various iron-inhibitors like polyphenols, phosvitin, and calcium. This recipe was provided by Inga Voloshin, RDN.

Yield: 4 (½-cup) servings   **Prep time:** 20 minutes
Cook time: 35 minutes

2 cups whole milk

½ vanilla bean, scraped

1 cinnamon stick

2 (1-inch) slices fresh ginger

¼ teaspoon whole black peppercorns

pinch of salt

3 tea bags black tea (Earl Grey or Lipton will do)

½ cup granulated sugar, divided

5 egg yolks

1. Place the milk, vanilla seeds and scraped bean, cinnamon stick, ginger, peppercorns, salt, tea bags, and ¼ cup sugar into a medium saucepan over low heat. Bring to a faint simmer, then remove from the heat. Discard the tea bags.

2. In a medium bowl, whisk the yolks with the remaining ¼ cup sugar. Gradually pour the hot milk mixture into the bowl, whisking continually. Return the mixture to the saucepan. Cook, stirring constantly, over very low heat for 3 to 4 minutes, until the mixture thickens slightly and coats the back of a wooden spoon.

3. Discard the spices, and strain the mixture into a medium bowl or container. Let cool to room temperature, and then continue to chill in the refrigerator for at least 1 hour.

4. Pour into an ice cream machine and churn according to manufacturer's instructions (my Cuisinart ice cream machine took 30 minutes). Transfer the churned ice cream to a freezer-safe container and chill in the freezer until ready to eat. If you can't wait that long, you will have to settle for soft-serve ice cream.

Nutrition facts per serving
245 calories | 9.7 g total fat | 4.3 g saturated fat | 32.3 g carbohydrate | 0.4 g fiber | 7.5 g protein | 0.63 mg iron | 174 mg calcium

Frozen Yogurt Cups

This delicious, sweet treat also makes for a super-satisfying breakfast.

Yield: 2 servings   **Prep time:** 10 minutes

  2 cups nonfat vanilla Greek yogurt

  1 cup sliced strawberries or berry of choice

1. Mix together the Greek yogurt and strawberries.

2. Pour the mixture into a lined muffin tin.

3. Freeze until solid, 1 to 2 hours. Enjoy frozen.

Nutrition facts per serving
216 calories | 0.5 g total fat | 0 g saturated fat | 33.5 g carbohydrate |
1.5 g fiber | 20.5 g protein | 0.36 mg iron | 15mg calcium

Pistachio Coconut Yogurt Pops

A frozen yogurt treat equipped with protein, probiotics, and flavor—that's something to get excited about! This recipe was provided by Inga Voloshin, RDN.

Yield: 8 servings
Prep time: 10 minutes, plus at least 6 hours to freeze

1 cup shelled pistachios	2 cups vanilla Greek yogurt
½ cup shredded coconut flakes	1 single-serve packet probiotic supplement (optional)

1. Pulse the pistachios and coconut flakes together in a food processor just until slightly broken up.

2. Add the yogurt and probiotic supplement, if using, and combine until everything is mixed thoroughly.

3. Distribute the mixture among eight Popsicle molds. Freeze overnight or for at least 6 hours.

4. To unmold, place the Popsicle molds under running hot water for a few seconds.

Nutrition facts per serving
311 calories | 23.7 g total fat | 9.9 g saturated fat | 18 g carbohydrate | 6 g fiber | 11 g protein | 1.1 mg iron | 70 mg calcium

Mocha Cookies

Delicious cookies that also happen to incorporate some iron-inhibiting polyphenols. This recipe was provided by Inga Voloshin, RDN.

Yield: About 12 cookies **Prep time:** 25 minutes plus 20 minutes to chill
Cook time: 12 minutes

1 stick unsalted butter

1 cup plus 2 tablespoons sugar, divided

1 egg

1 teaspoon espresso powder (or instant coffee), dissolved in 1 tablespoon hot water

1 teaspoon vanilla extract

1 cup all-purpose flour

¼ cup plus 2 teaspoons unsweetened cocoa powder, divided

1 teaspoon baking soda

1 teaspoon baking powder

⅛ teaspoon ground cinnamon

⅛ teaspoon salt

1. Preheat the oven to 375°F. Line two rectangular half (18 x 13-inch) sheet pans with parchment paper.

2. In a large bowl or an electric mixer fitted with a paddle attachment, cream the butter and 1 cup sugar until pale yellow and creamy. Continue to mix as you add the egg, espresso solution, and vanilla extract.

3. In a separate bowl, combine the flour, ¼ cup cocoa powder, baking soda, baking powder, cinnamon, and salt. Add the flour mixture to the butter mixture, and mix until combined. Chill the cookie batter in the refrigerator for 20 minutes.

4. In a small bowl, combine the remaining 2 teaspoons of cocoa powder with the 2 tablespoons of sugar, and set aside.

5. Roll the chilled cookie batter into balls (slightly smaller than the size of a golf ball), dip into the cocoa-sugar mixture, and place on the sheet pan, making sure to provide 2 inches between each cookie.

6. Bake about 12 minutes until the cookies are still soft to the touch. Let stand 5 minutes before removing from pan.

Nutrition facts per serving
149 calories | 8 g total fat | 5 g saturated fat | 19.9 g carbohydrate | 0.8 g fiber | 1 g protein | 0.4 mg iron | 70 mg calcium

Brown Rice Pudding

Who doesn't love a healthy spin on a favorite classic dessert? This version incorporates a whole grain, is lower in fat, and goes lighter on the sugar. Not only is this combination overall healthier, it also has more of an inhibitory effect on iron than the original.

Yield: 8 servings   **Prep time:** 5 minutes
Cook time: 40 minutes

1 cup jasmine brown rice

2 cups water

pinch of salt

2 cups low-fat milk

4 ounces evaporated fat-free milk

½ teaspoon vanilla extract

1 teaspoon ground cinnamon

¼ cup sugar

1. Place the brown rice into a medium saucepan with the water and a pinch of salt.

2. Bring the rice to a boil over medium-high heat.

3. Once boiling, cover with a lid and reduce the heat to medium-low.

4. Let the rice simmer for approximately 25 minutes, or until all of the water has been absorbed.

5. Once the rice is done, pour in the low-fat milk, evaporated milk, vanilla extract, cinnamon, and sugar. Stir well.

6. Simmer uncovered over low heat for about 10 to 15 minutes, stirring often, until it thickens.

7. Enjoy warm or cold.

Nutrition facts per serving
143 calories | 0.6 g total fat | 0.4 g saturated fat | 30.1 g carbohydrate | 0.7 g fiber | 4 g protein | 0.02 mg iron | 105 mg calcium

Apple Chips

Another way to enjoy fruit between meals is in the form of chips. With minimal ingredients, you can create the perfect snack for when you are on the go!

Yield: 4 servings   **Prep time:** 25 minutes   **Cook time:** 2 to 2½ hours

4 large Pink Lady or Honeycrisp apples, cored and thinly sliced with a mandolin

1 teaspoon ground cinnamon

¼ teaspoon ginger powder

1. Preheat the oven to 200°F.

2. On two parchment paper–lined baking (18 x 13-inch) half sheet pans, place the apple slices in a single layer.

3. Lightly sprinkle the apple slices with the cinnamon and ginger. If you have any of the seasonings left, flip the slices over and sprinkle the other side.

4. Bake in the oven for 1 hour. Flip the apples and then return to the oven for another 1 to 1½ hours, until crispy.

5. Once crispy, allow the apples to sit on the stovetop for 5 minutes. If after this point they aren't crispy enough, bake them a little longer.

6. Once finished, allow the apple slices to cool prior to enjoying or storing them in an airtight container for up to 1 week.

Nutrition facts per serving
112 calories | 0.4 g total fat | 0.1 g saturated fat | 31.3 g carbohydrate | 5.7 g fiber | 0.6 g protein | 0.22 mg iron | 16 mg calcium

Banana Soft Serve

On a hot summer day, you might find yourself torn between having a serving of fruit at snack time and wanting a cup of ice cream or frozen yogurt. To end the struggle, turn to this "nice-cream"—who says you can't have your cake and eat it too?!

Yield: 2 servings   **Prep time:** 5 minutes

2 ripe bananas, frozen

½ cup unsweetened vanilla almond milk or low-fat milk

¼ teaspoon ground cinnamon

Place all ingredients into a blender. Blend until creamy but thick. If it's ice cream you're after, then simply freeze for a half hour before serving. Enjoy!

Nutrition facts per serving
122 calories | 0.7 g total fat | 0 g saturated fat | 30.3 g carbohydrate | 5.3 g fiber | 1.4 g protein | 0.45 mg iron | 148 mg calcium

Conversions

VOLUME

U.S.	U.S. EQUIVALENT	METRIC
1 tablespoon (3 teaspoons)	½ fluid ounce	15 milliliters
¼ cup	2 fluid ounces	60 milliliters
⅓ cup	3 fluid ounces	80 milliliters
½ cup	4 fluid ounces	120 milliliters
⅔ cup	5 fluid ounces	160 milliliters
¾ cup	6 fluid ounces	180 milliliters
1 cup	8 fluid ounces	240 milliliters
2 cups	16 fluid ounces	480 milliliters

WEIGHT

U.S.	METRIC
½ ounce	15 grams
1 ounce	30 grams
2 ounces	60 grams
¼ pound	115 grams
⅓ pound	150 grams
½ pound	225 grams
¾ pound	340 grams
1 pound	450 grams

TEMPERATURE

FAHRENHEIT (°F)	CELSIUS (°C)	FAHRENHEIT (°F)	CELSIUS (°C)
70°F	20°C	240°F	115°C
100°F	40°C	260°F	125°C
120°F	50°C	280°F	140°C
130°F	55°C	300°F	150°C
140°F	60°C	325°F	165°C
150°F	65°C	350°F	175°C
160°F	70°C	375°F	190°C
170°F	75°C	400°F	200°C
180°F	80°C	425°F	220°C
190°F	90°C	450°F	230°C
200°F	95°C	500°F	260°C
220°F	105°C		

References

Abbaspour, Nazanin, Richard Hurrell, and Roya Kelishadi. "Review on Iron and Its Importance for Human Health." *Journal of Research in Medical Sciences* 19 (2014): 164–174.

Acton, Ronald T. and Barton C. James. "Diabetes in HFE Hemochromatosis." *Journal of Diabetes Research* (February 2017): 1–16. https://doi.org/10.1155/2017/9826930.

"Alcohol: How Much Is Safe—In the Presence of Excess Iron?" *Iron Disorders Institute nanograms* (February 2011).

Aranda, Núria, Fernando E. Viteri, Carme Montserrat, and Victoria Arija. "Effects of C282Y, H63D, and S65C HFE Gene Mutations, Diet, and Lifestyle Factors on Iron Status in a General Mediterranean Population from Tarragona, Spain." *Annals of Hematology* 89, no. 8 (2010): 767–773. https://doi.org/10.1007/s00277-010-0901-9.

"Are Eggs Good for You or Not?" www.heart.org. Accessed April 1, 2019. https://www.heart.org/en/news/2018/08/15/are-eggs-good-for-you-or-not.

Arezes, João, Grace Jung, Victoria Gabayan, Erika Valore, Piotr Ruchala, Paul A. Gulig, Tomas Ganz, Elizabeta Nemeth, and Yonca Bulut. "Hepcidin-Induced Hypoferremia Is a Critical Host Defense Mechanism against the Siderophilic Bacterium Vibrio Vulnificus." *Cell Host & Microbe* 17, no. 1 (2015): 47–57. https://doi:10.1016/j.chom.2014.12.001.

Bacon, Bruce R., Paul C. Adams, Kris V. Kowdley, Lawrie W. Powell, and Anthony S. Tavill."Diagnosis and Management of Hemochromatosis: 2011 Practice Guideline by the American Association for the Study of Liver Diseases." *Hepatology* 54, no. 1 (2011): 328–343. https://doi.org/10.1002/hep.24330.

Bacon, Bruce R., Stanley L. Schrier, and Janet L. Kwiatkowski. "Patient Education: Hereditary Hemochromatosis (Beyond the Basics)." UpToDate. (January 2019). https://www.uptodate.com/contents/hereditary-hemochromatosis-beyond-the-basics?search=iron%20overload&source=search_result&selectedTitle=2~150&usage_type=default&display_rank=2.

Badria, Farid A., Ahmed S. Ibrahim, Adel F. Badria, and Ahmed A. Elmarakby. "Curcumin Attenuates Iron Accumulation and Oxidative Stress in the Liver and Spleen of Chronic Iron-Overloaded Rats." *Plos One* 10, no. 7 (2015) 1–13. https://doi.org/10.1371/journal.pone.0134156.

Barton, James C., Corwin Q. Edwards, Pradyumna D. Phatak. Britton, Robert S., and Bruce R. Bacon. "Complications of Hemochromatosis and Iron Overload" in *Handbook of Iron Overload Disorders*. New York: Cambridge University Press, 2010.

Bataller, Ramón. "Time to Ban Smoking in Patients with Chronic Liver Diseases." *Hepatology* 44, no. 6 (2006): 1394–396. https://doi:10.1002/hep.21484.

Bonsmann, Storcksdieck, T. Walczyk, S. Renggli, and R. F. Hurrell. "Oxalic Acid Does Not Influence Nonhaem Iron Absorption in Humans: A Comparison of Kale and Spinach Meals." *European Journal of Clinical Nutrition* 62 (2008): 336–341. https://doi.org/10.1038/sj.ejcn.1602721.

Bovenschen, H. Jorn and Wynand HPM Vissers. "Primary Hemochromatosis Presented by Porphyria Cutanea Tarda: A Case Report." *Cases Journal* 2, no. 7246 (2009): 1–4. doi: 10.4076/1757-1626-2-7246.

Camacho, Antonio, Thomas Funck-Brentano, Marcio Simao, Leonor Cancela, Sebastien Ottaviani, Martine Cohen-Solal, and Pascal Richette. "Effect of C282Y Genotype on Self-Reported Musculoskeletal Complications in Hereditary Hemochromatosis." *Plos One*, no. 3 (2015): 1–8. https://doi.org/10.1371/journal.pone.0122817.

Carr, Anitra and Margreet C. M. Vissers. "Synthetic or Food-Derived Vitamin C—Are They Equally Bioavailable?" *Nutrients* 5, no. 11 (2013): 4284–4304. https://doi.org/10.3390/nu5114284.

Chai, Weiswen and Michael Liebman. "Effect of Different Cooking Methods on Vegetable Oxalate Content." *Journal of Agricultural and Food Chemistry* 53, no. 8 (2005): 3027–3030.

"Chapter 1 Key Elements of Healthy Eating Patterns." A Closer Look Inside Healthy Eating Patterns 2015–2020 Dietary Guidelines. Accessed April 01, 2019. https://health.gov/dietaryguidelines/2015/guidelines/chapter-1/a-closer-look-inside-healthy-eating-patterns.

Christides, Tatiana and Paul Sharp. "Sugars Increase Non-Heme Iron Bioavailability in Human Epithelial Intestinal and Liver Cells." *Plos One* 8, no. 12 (2013): 1–8. https://doi.org/10.1371/journal.pone.0083031.

"Cirrhosis of the Liver." American Liver Foundation. Accessed March 28, 2019. https://liverfoundation.org/for-patients/about-the-liver/diseases-of-the-liver/cirrhosis/#information-for-the-newly-diagnosed.

"Classic Hereditary Hemochromatosis." National Organization for Rare Disorders. Accessed March 28, 2019. https://rarediseases.org/rare-diseases/classic-hereditary-hemochromatosis.

Condrasky, Margaret D. and M. Hegler. "Lingering Tannins." *Culinary Nutrition News* (2012): 1–2.

Dallow, Tomas, Enijad Sahinbegovic, et al. "Idiopathic Hand Osteoarthritis vs. Haemochromatosis Arthropathy—A Clinical, Functional and Radiographic Study." *Rheumatology* (2013): 910–915. doi:10.1093/rheumatology/kes392.

Dejaco, Christian, Andreas Stadlmayr, et al. "Ultrasound Verified Inflammation and Structural Damage in Patients with Hereditary Haemochromatosis-Related Arthropathy." *Arthritis Research & Therapy* 19, no. 243 (2017): 1–10. doi:10.1186/s13075-017-1448-0.

Delimont, Nicole M., Mark D. Haub, and Brian L. Lindshield. "The Impact of Tannin Consumption on Iron Bioavailability and Status: A Narrative Review." *Current Developments in Nutrition* (2017): 1–12. https://doi.org/10.3945/cdn.116.000042.

Fleming, Diana J., Katherine L. Tucker, et al. "Dietary Factors Associated with the Risk of High Iron Stores in the Elderly Framingham Heart Study Cohort." *The American Journal of Clinical Nutrition* 76 (2002): 1375–1384.

Fleming, Diana J., Paul F. Jacques, et al. "Dietary Determinants of Iron Stores in a Free-Living Elderly Population: The Framingham Heart Study." *American Journal of Clinical Nutrition* 67 (1998): 722–733.

Fletcher, Linda M., Kim R. Bridle, and Darrell H. G. Crawford. "Effect of Alcohol on Iron Storage Diseases of the Liver." *Best Practice & Research Clinical Gastroenterology* 17, no. 4 (2003): 663–677. https://doi:10.1053/ybega.2003.378.

"Food Sources of Vitamin C." *Dietitians of Canada* (2015). Accessed April 01, 2019. https://www.dietitians.ca/getattachment/c15a51ce-ab6c-4c46-bac3-924e8e213e6b/Factsheet-Food-Sources-of-Vitamin-C.pdf.aspx.

Fraietta, Renato, Daniel S., Zylberstein, and Sandro C. Esteves. "Hypogonadotropic Hypogonadism Revisited." *Clinics* 68, no. 1 (2013): 81–88. doi: 10.6061/clinics/2013(Sup01)09.

Garrison, Cheryl. *The Iron Disorders Institute Guide to Hemochromatosis*. Naperville, IL: Cumberland House, 2009.

Gautam, Smita, Kalpana Platel, and Krishnapura Srinivasan. "Influence of B-carotene-rich Vegetables on the Bioaccessibility of Zinc and Iron from Food Grains." *Food Chemistry* 122 (2010): 668–672.

GBD 2016 Alcohol Collaborators. "Alcohol Use and Burden for 195 Countries and Territories, 1990-2016: A Systemic Analysis for the Global Burden of Disease Study 2016." *The Lancet* 392 (2018): 1015–1035. http://doi.org/10.1016/S0140-6736(18)31310-2.

Geller, Stephen A. and Fernando P. F. de Campos. "Hereditary Hemochromatosis." *Autopsy & Case Reports* 5, no. 1 (2015): 7–10. doi: 10.4322/acr.2014.043.

Girelli, Domenico, Elizabeta Nemeth, and Dorine W. Swinkels. "Hepcidin in the Diagnosis of Iron Disorders." *Blood* 127, no. 23 (2015): 2809–13. https://doi.org/10.1182/blood-2015-12-639112.

Gropper, Sareen S., Jack L. Smith, and James L. Groff. "Microminerals" in *Advanced Nutrition and Human Metabolism Fifth Edition*, 470-487. Belmont: Wadsworth Cengage Learning, 2009.

Grosse, Scott D. and Muin J. Khoury. "A New Public Health Assessment of the Disease Burden of Hereditary Hemochromatosis: How Clinically Actionable is C282Y Homozygosity?" Centers for Disease Control and Prevention (August 2017). Accessed March 31, 2019. https://blogs.cdc.gov/genomics/2017/08/16/a-new-public-health-assessment/.

Gujja, Pradeep, Douglas R., Rosing, Dorothy J. Tripodi, and Yukitaka Shizukuda. "Iron Overload Cardiomyopathy, Better Understanding of an Increasing Disorder." *Journal of the American College of Cardiology* 56, no. 13 (September 2011): 1001–1012. doi:10.1016/j.jacc.2010.03.083.

Gupta, Sheetal, Jothi A. Lakshmi, and Jamuna Prakash. "In Vitro Bioavailability of Calcium and Iron from Selected Green Lady Vegetables." *Journal of the Science of Food and Agriculture* 86 (2006): 2147–2152. https://doi.org/10.1002/jsfa.2589.

Hagström, Hannes. "Alcohol Consumption in Concomitant Liver Disease: How Much Is Too Much?" *Current Hepatology Reports* 16, no. 2 (2017): 152–157. doi:10.1007/s11901-017-0343-0.

Halberg, Leif and Lena Hulthen. "Prediction of Dietary Absorption: an Algorithm for Calculating Absorption and Bioavailability of Dietary Iron." *American Journal of Clinical Nutrition* 71 (2000): 1147–1160.

Hallberg, Leif and Lena Hulthen. "Prediction of Dietary Iron Absorption: An Algorithm for Calculating Absorption and Bioavailability of Dietary Iron. *American Journal of Clinical Nutrition* 17, no. 1 (2000): 1147–1160.

"Health Effects." Smokefree.gov. Accessed April 01, 2019. https://smoke-free.gov/quit-smoking/why-you-should-quit/health-effects.

"Hemochromatosis and Cardiomyopathy." Cardiomyopathy UK. April 2017. Accessed March 28, 2019. https://www.cardiomyopathy.org/about-cardiomyopathy/haemochromatosis-and-cardiomyopathy.

"Hemochromatosis Type 1." National Institutes of Health. Accessed March 28, 2019, https://rarediseases.info.nih.gov/diseases/10417/hemochromatosis-type-1.

Hemochromatosis, Type 1." Human Phenotype Ontology. Accessed March 28, 2019, https://hpo.jax.org/app/browse/disease/OMIM:235200.

"Hemochromatosis." *National Digestive Diseases Information Clearinghouse*, no. 14-4621 (2014): 1–8.

"Hemochromatosis." National Institutes of Health. Accessed March 28, 2019, https://rarediseases.info.nih.gov/diseases/10746/hemochromatosis.

Hernando, Diego, Yakir S. Levin, Calude B. Sirlin, and Scott B. Reeder. "Quantification of Liver Iron with MRI: State of the Art and Remaining Challenges." *Journal of Magnetic Resonance Imaging* 40, no. 5 (2014): 1003–1021. https://doi: 10.1002/jmri.24584.

Hewlings, Susan J. and Douglas S. Kalman. "Curcumin: A Review of Its Effects on Human Health." *Foods* 6, no. 92 (2017): 1–11. https://www.nvbi.nlm.nih.gov.

"HFE Gene." National Institutes of Health. Accessed January 4, 2019. https://ghr.nlm.nih.gov/gene/HFE#conditions.

"How Does Skin Work?" InformedHealth.org and Institute for Quality and Efficiency in Health Care (IQWiG). July 28, 2016. Accessed March 28, 2019. https://www.ncbi.nlm.nih.gov/pubmedhealth/PMH0072439.

"How Does the Pancreas Work?" InformedHealth.org and Institute for Quality and Efficiency in Health Care. (September 2018). Accessed March 28, 2019. https://www.ncbi.nlm.nih.gov/pubmedhealth/PMH0072490.

Hurrell, Richard and Ines Egli. "Iron Bioavailability and Dietary Reference Values." *The American Journal of Clinical Nutrition* 91 (2010): 1461S–1467S.

"Hypothalamus: MedlinePlus Medical Encyclopedia." MedlinePlus. May 21, 2017. Accessed March 31, 2019. https://medlineplus.gov/ency/article/002380.htm.

"Iron-Deficiency Anemia." National Heart Lung and Blood Institute. Accessed April 01, 2019. https://www.nhlbi.nih.gov/health-topics/iron-deficiency-anemia.

Ishikawa, S. I., S. Tamaki, K. Arihara, and M. Itoh. "Egg Yolk Protein and Egg Yolk Phosvitin Inhibit Calcium, Magnesium, and Iron Absorption in Rats." *Journal of Food Science* 72, no. 6 (2007): S412–S419. https://doi.org/10.1111/j.1750-3841.2007.00417.x.

Kim, Hyungjo, Chol Shin, and Inkyung Baik. "Associations Between Lifestyle Factors and Iron Overload in Korean Adults." *Clinical Nutrition Research* 5, no. 4 (2016): 270–278. https://doi.org/10.7762/cnr.2016.5.4.270.

Kim, Kyung H. and Ki Young Oh. "Clinical Applications of Therapeutic Phlebotomy." *Journal of Blood Medicine* 7 (2016): 139–144. https://doi:10.2147/JBM.S108479.

Lamy, Elsa, Cristina Pinheiro, Lenia Rodrigues, Fernando Capela e Silva, Orlando Silvia Lopes, Sofia Tavares, and Rui Gaspar. "Determinants of Tannin-Rich Food and Beverage Consumption: Oral Perception vs. Psychosocial Aspects" in *Tannins: Biochemistry, Food Sources, and Nutritional Properties*. Combs, CA: Nova Science Publishers Inc., 2016.

Lans, Jonathan, Jacques A. Machol, et al. "Nonrheumatoid Arthritis of the Hand." *The Journal of Hand Surgery* volume 43, no. 1 (2018): 61–67. https://doi.org/10.1016/j.jhsa.2017.10.021.

Leider, Morris. "On the Weight of the Skin." *The Journal of Investigative Dermatology*. (November 1948): 187–191.

Leitman, Susan F. "Hemochromatosis: The New Blood Donor." *American Society of Hematology* (2013): 645–650.

"Living with Hepatitis: How to Stay Healthy." DC.gov. Accessed March 31, 2019. https://dchealth.dc.gov/service/living-hepatitis-how-stay-healthy.

Lotfield, Erikka, Neal D. Freedman, et al. "Association of Coffee Consumption with Overall and Cause-Specific Mortality in a Large US Prospective Cohort Study. *American Journal of Epidemiology* 182, no. 12 (2015): 1010–1022. https://doi.org/10.1093/aje/kwv146.

Mascitelli, L. and M. R. Goldstein. "Inhibition of Iron Absorption by Polyphenols as an Anti-cancer Mechanism." *Qjm* 104, no. 5 (2010): 459–461. https://doi.org/10.1093/qjmed/hcq239.

Meatless Monday. Accessed April 01, 2019. https://www.meatlessmonday.com.

Milstone, Leonard M., Rong-Hua Hu, et al. "Impact of Epidermal Desquamation on Tissue Stores of Iron." *Journal of Dermatological Science* 67, no. 1 (2012): 9–14. doi: 10.1016/j.jdermsci.2012.04.003.

Milward, Elizabeth A., Surinder K. Baines, et al. "Noncitrus Fruits as Novel Dietary Environmental Modifiers of Iron Stores in People With or Without HFE Gene Mutations." *Mayo Clinic Proceedings* 83, no. 5 (2008): 543–49. https://doi.org/10.4065/835543.

Mobarra, Naser, Mehrnoosh Shanaki, et al. "A Review on Iron Chelators in Treatment of Iron Overload Syndromes." *International Journal of Hematology-Oncology and Stem Cell Research* 10, no. 4 (2016): 239–247.

Moore, Marisa. "How Vitamin C Supports a Healthy Immune System." Eatright. Academy of Nutrition and Dietetics. December 21, 2016. Accessed January 05, 2019. https://www.eatright.org/food/vitamins-and-supplements/types-of-vitamins-and-nutrients/how-vitamin-c-supports-a-healthy-immune-system.

Nemeth, Elizabeta and Tomas Ganz. "The Role of Hepcidin in Iron Metabolism." *Acta Haematologica* 122, no. 2–3 (November 2009): 78–86. doi: 10.1159/000243791.

"Office of Dietary Supplements—Calcium." NIH Office of Dietary Supplements. Accessed April 01, 2019. https://ods.od.nih.gov/factsheets/Calcium-HealthProfessional.

Pavenski, Katerina. "Therapeutic Apheresis." Canadian Blood Services. August 01, 2018. Accessed March 31, 2019. https://professionaleducation.blood.ca/en/transfusion/clinical-guide/therapeutic-apheresis.

Pedersen, Palle and Nils Milman. "Extrinsic Factors Modifying Expressivity of the HFE Variant C282Y, H63D, S65C Phenotypes in 1,294 Danish Men." *Annals of Hematology* 88 (2009): 957–965. https://doi.org/10.1007/s00277-009-0714-x.

Quibntaes, K. D., A. Cilla and R. Barbera. "Iron Bioavailability from Cereal Foods Fortified with Iron." *Austin Journal of Nutrition & Metabolism* 2, no. 3 (2015): 1–9.

Reisdorf, Ana G. "Beauty and Nutrition—Evidence-Based Dietary Practices Can Help Patients Look and Feel Their Best." *Today's Dietitian* 18, no. 9 (2016): 56.

Rigas, Andreas S., Benedikte H. Ejsing, et al. "Calcium in Drinking Water: Effect on Iron Stores in Danish Blood Donors—Results from the Danish Blood Donor Study." *Transfusion* 58, no. 6 (2018): 1468–473. https://doi.org/10.1111/trf.14600.

Rombout-Sestrienkova, Eva, Marian G. J. van Kraaij, and Ger H. Koek. "How We Manage Patients with Hereditary Haemochromatosis." *British Journal of Haematology* 175 (2016): 759–770. https://doi.org/10.1111/bjh.14376.

Samman, Samir. "Iron." *Nutrition & Dietetics* 64, no. S4 (2007): S126–S130. https://doi:10.1111/j.1747-0080.2007.00199.x.

Scheckel, Kristen A. and Ravin J. Mehta. "Hereditary Hemochromatosis as a Cause of Hypogonadism." *Clinician Reviews* (2013): 26–33.

Schlemmer, Ulrich, Wenche Frolich, Rafel M. Prieto, and Felix Grases. "Phytate in Foods and Significance for Humans: Food Sources, Intake, Processing, Bioavailability, Protective Role and Analysis." *Molecular Nutrition Food Research* 53 (2009): S330–S375. https://doi.org/10.1002/mnfr.200900099.

Schepers, Anastasia. "Concerned About Your Cookware? EN Answers Common Questions." *Environmental Nutrition 23, no.* 5 (2000): 2. Accessed April 01, 2019. http://link.galegroup.com.proxy.wexler.hunter.cuny.edu/apps/doc/A62302741/HRCA?u=cuny_hunter&sid=HRCA&xid=94543e89.

Sizer, Frances S., Eleanor Noss Whitney, and Leonard A. Piche. *Nutrition: Concepts and Controversies.* Toronto: Nelson Education, 2012.

Stubblefield, Carol. "Haemochromatosis and Raw Oysters: a Dangerous Combination." *Australian Nursing Journal* 3, no. 4 (1995): 36–37.

Sundic, Tatjana, Tor Hervig, et al. "Erythrocytapheresis Compared with Whole Blood Phlebotomy Treatment of Hereditary Haemochromatosis." *Blood Transfusion* 12 (2014): S84–89. https://doi.org/10.2450/2013.0128-13.

"Symptoms." Canadian Hemochromatosis Society. Accessed March 28, 2019, https://www.toomuchiron.ca/hemochromatosis/symptoms.

Tavill, Anthony S. "Hemochromatosis." The Cleveland Clinic Foundation. (August 2017). Accessed March 31, 2019. http://www.cleveland-clinicmeded.com/medicalpubs/diseasemanagement/hepatology/hemochromatosis.

US Preventative Services Task Force. "Screening for Hemochromatosis: Recommendation Statement." *Annals of Internal Medicine* 145, no. 3 (2006): 204–208.

Van Doorn, Gerdien and Irene Gosselink. *Dietary Advice in HFE-hemochromatosis.* May 2012.

"Vitamin C." American Optometric Association. Accessed April 01, 2019. https://www.aoa.org/patients-and-public/caring-for-your-vision/diet-and-nutrition/vitamin-c.

"Vitamin C." *The Nutrition Source*. Accessed April 01, 2019. https://www.hsph.harvard.edu/nutritionsource/vitamin-c.

"Vitamin C (Ascorbic Acid): Uses, Side Effects, Interactions, Dosage, and Warning." WebMD. Accessed April 01, 2019. https://www.webmd.com/vitamins/ai/ingredientmono-1001/vitamin-c-ascorbic-acid.

Vucenik, I. and AbulKalam M. Shamsuddin. "Protection Against Cancer by Dietary IP6 and Inositol." *Nutrition and Cancer* 55, no. 2 (2006): 109–125. https://doi.org/10.1207/s15327914nc5502_1.

Walker-Esbaugh, Cheryl, Laine H. McCarthy, and Rhonda A. Sparks. *Dunmore and Fleischer's Medical Terminology: Exercises in Etymology*, 3rd Edition. Philadelphia, PA: F. A. Davis Company, 2004.

Webb, Densie. "Antioxidants: The Carotenoid Color Wheel." *Today's Dietitian* 18, no. 9 (2016): 12. https://www.todaysdietitian.com/newarchives/0916p12.shtml.

Whalen, Nancy L. and John K. Olynyk. "Association of Transferring Saturation with the Arthropathy of Hereditary Hemochromatosis." *Clinical Gastroenterology and Hepatology* 15, no. 10 (2017): 1507–1508. http://dx.doi.org/10.1016/j.cgh.2017.06.018.

Whitlock, Evelyn P., Betsy A. Garlitz, et al. "Screening for Hereditary Hemochromatosis: A Systematic Review for the US Preventive Services Task Force." *Annals of Internal Medicine*. August 01, 2006. https://annals.org/aim/fullarticle/726823/screening-hereditary-hemochromatosis-sys-tematic-review-u-s-preventive-services-task.

Yadav, S. K., and S. Sehgal. "Effect of Domestic Processing and Cooking Methods on Total, HCL Extractable Iron and In Vitro Availability of Iron in Spinach and Amaranth Leaves." *Nutrition and Health* 16 (2002): 113–120.

Zakko, Liam, Justin Finch, Marti J. Rothe, and Jane M. Grant-Kels. "Hemochromatosis: Dermatological Features." *Atlas of Dermatological Manifestations of Gastrointestinal Disease*. New York: Springer Science + Business Media, 2013.

Recipe Index

Acknowledgments

It is with immense gratitude that I wish to acknowledge the following people for their support throughout my journey of writing this book:

My mother, Inna Khesin, for devoting countless hours to helping me test my recipe creations and reporting back with constructive feedback. For always believing in me and showering me with love and encouragement.

My father, Alexander Khesin, for always being the eager and willing recipe taster. For believing in me and pushing me to go after opportunities that help me grow and evolve.

My partner in life, Dr. Mark Kreimer, for offering continuous encouragement and dedicating many late hours to reading early drafts and providing invaluable input.

My friend, fellow dietitian and recipe contributor, Inga Voloshin, RDN, for being the mastermind behind the Pistachio Coconut Yogurt Pops (page 119), Chai Tea Ice Cream (page 116), and Mocha Cookies (page 120) recipes. Prior to becoming a dietitian, Inga received her degree in the culinary arts at the Institute of Culinary Education, which led her to explore a passion for cooking and food by working in some of New York City's finest catering establishments and restaurants. She has since fused her love of the culinary arts and nutrition in her latest blog, Hungry-Healthy.com.

The team at Ulysses Press, especially my editors Casie Vogel and Renee Rutledge, for helping to make this book a reality.

Last but not least, my entire family and dear friends for being my biggest cheerleaders.

About the Author

Anna Khesin, RD, CDN, is a registered dietitian and certified dietitian nutritionist on a mission to awaken an appetite for healthy living in others. Her experience spans clinical, corporate, private, and community settings, and has led to a keen interest in disease states in which nutrition plays an important role.

Anna counsels a wide array of patients in a private practice setting in Edgewater, New Jersey. She graduated from Queens College with a bachelor's degree in family and consumer sciences and completed her dietetic internship through Long Island University Post campus. Anna lives in North Bergen, New Jersey.